T0255726

Quick Reference Dictionary FOR Orthopedics

Edited by

Antonia F. Chen, MD, MBA
University of Pittsburgh
Department of Orthopaedic Surgery
Pittsburgh, Pennsylvania

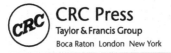

CRC Press
Taylor & Francis Group
Boca Raton London New York

CRC Press is an imprint of the
Taylor & Francis Group, an **informa** business

Dr. Antonia F. Chen receives grant support from the Orthopaedic Research Educational Foundation, The Pittsburgh Foundation, and the Scoliosis Research Society.

Illustrations by Emily Benson unless otherwise referenced.

First published 2012 by SLACK Incorporated

Published 2024 by CRC Press
2385 NW Executive Center Drive, Suite 320, Boca Raton FL 33431

and by CRC Press
4 Park Square, Milton Park, Abingdon, Oxon, OX14 4RN

CRC Press is an imprint of Taylor & Francis Group, LLC

© 2012 Taylor & Francis Group, LLC

Library of Congress Cataloging-in-Publication Data

Quick reference dictionary for orthopedics / edited by Antonia Chen.
   p. ; cm.
 Includes bibliographical references and index.
 ISBN 978-1-55642-989-7 (alk. paper)
 I. Chen, Antonia.
 [DNLM: 1. Orthopedics--Dictionary--English. WE 13]

 616.7003--dc23

                         2012012558

ISBN: 9781556429897 (pbk)
ISBN: 9781003526186 (ebk)

DOI: 10.1201/9781003526186

Dedication

This book is dedicated to my mother, Dr. Jean F. Lian, who raised me and has always believed in me. Without her love, support, strength, and courage, I would not be the woman and doctor that I am today.

This book is also dedicated to my sister, Victoria F. Chen, who always cheers me on, who always has my back, and who always has a listening ear. Thank you for being one of my biggest supporters.

To my friends and mentors in orthopedics, Dr. Brian A. Klatt and Dr. Alfred J. Tria Jr, both of whom inspired me, taught me, and encouraged me to become an academic arthroplasty surgeon.

Finally, this book is dedicated to my significant other, Dr. MingDe Lin, who edited this *Quick Reference Dictionary* countless times, who keeps me grounded, who supports me in all my crazy endeavors, and who shows unconditional love.

Contents

Acknowledgments

This book was only made possible with the help and influence of many individuals. First of all, I would like to thank the following individuals at SLACK Incorporated: Carrie Kotlar, John Bond, and April Billick, whose support and guidance made this book possible. I would also like to thank Dr. Emily Benson for her patience and her amazing illustrations. Thank you to Dr. Brian A. Klatt for suggesting that I take on this project.

Personally, I would like to thank Dr. Bor-Kuan Chen for his scientific advice and influence in my life. I would also like to thank Dr. Wenmin Chuu for providing guidance and support to our family.

Professionally, I would like to thank Dr. Freddie H. Fu for being my role model, my chairman, and a great educator. I would also like to thank Dr. Alfred J. Tria, who inspired me to pursue a career in orthopedics. My sincere thanks to Dr. Lawrence S. Crossett and Dr. Adolph "Chick" Yates for being outstanding arthroplasty surgeons who have patiently taught me and guided me. Thank you to Dr. Nalini Rao for the many projects we have pursued together and for piquing my interest in periprosthetic infections. Additionally, I would like to thank Dr. Rocky S. Tuan for believing in me and encouraging me to pursue research. I would also like to thank Dr. Jonathan H. Waters for collaborating on projects and for being a mentor in blood management.

Many individuals within the Department of Orthopedics at the University of Pittsburgh have greatly influenced my education during my orthopedic residency and I thank them from the bottom of my heart. These individuals include Dr. Lance M. Brunton, Dr. Vincent F. X. Deeney, Dr. William F. Donaldson, Dr. Andrew R. Evans, Dr. David P. Fowler, Dr. Mark A. Goodman, Dr. Jan S. Grudziak, Dr. Gary S. Gruen,

Dr. Christopher D. Harner, Dr. James D. Kang, Dr. Robert A. Kaufmann, Dr. Joon Y. Lee, Dr. Richard L. McGough III, Dr. Stephen A. Mendelson, Dr. Volker Musahl, Dr. Victor R. Prisk, Dr. James W. Roach, Dr. Michael J. Rogal, Dr. Peter A. Siska, Dr. Ivan S. Tarkin, Dr. W. Timothy Ward, Dr. Kurt R. Weiss, Dr. Dane K. Wukich, and Dr. Vonda J. Wright.

To all of my attendings, fellow residents, and medical students I have worked with—thank you for your dedication to the field, for teaching me, and for being current and future colleagues.

For my friends and family—thank you for your unwavering support; it means the world to me.

About the Editor

Antonia F. Chen, MD, MBA received her bachelor of science degree from Yale University. She then received her medical degree from UMDNJ–Robert Wood Johnson, where she graduated with Distinction in Research and was inducted into the Alpha Omega Alpha Medical Honor Society. Antonia also received her master of business administration degree from Rutgers Business School and graduated as a member of the Beta Gamma Sigma Honor Society. She is currently an orthopedic resident at the University of Pittsburgh. In addition to clinical duties, her research interests are in arthroplasty and periprosthetic joint infections; she has delivered many podium presentations and posters on the national stage. Antonia has also received numerous awards during residency, including research awards and the Gold Foundation Humanism and Excellence in Teaching Award. She has served as a resident liaison for the membership committee in the American Association of Hip and Knee Surgeons. Antonia hopes to pursue a rewarding career as an academic arthroplasty surgeon.

Preface

I remember the first day of my orthopedic rotation. My pockets were filled to the brim with various books that covered anatomy, fracture classifications, and surgical approaches. Despite having all of these resources on hand, I realized that what I needed most was a pocket-sized dictionary to define all of the unfamiliar orthopedic terms being used. As I went on to residency, I realized that I needed a single, small reference book that contained all of the pertinent information relevant to the clinical care of orthopedic patients. This *Quick Reference Dictionary for Orthopedics* combines the best of both worlds—it is a dictionary that defines high-yield orthopedic terms, and contains appendices vital to managing orthopedic patients and navigating the field of orthopedics. It is a vital resource to be used on the wards and for any individual who has exposure to orthopedics.

Introduction

This book was created as an orthopedic reference tool for any individual who works within the field of orthopedics, specifically residents, medical students, nurses, and physical and occupational therapists. It is a comprehensive dictionary with over 2200 terms specific to orthopedics. The terms that are identified include muscle and bone anatomic descriptions, surgical techniques, syndromes, medications, surgical instruments, statistics terms, and more. Additionally, antonyms and synonyms are identified for certain terms. Finally, abbreviations are also provided that correlate with Appendix 1.

The appendices are unique as well, with each appendix highlighting a specific area relevant to orthopedics. Appendix 1 contains frequently used acronyms and abbreviations in orthopedics, many of which are used on a regular basis in progress notes, in surgery, or in conversation. Appendix 2 provides medical root terminology that serves as the basis of many commonly used terms. Appendices 3 through 7 cover anatomic descriptions, including terms (Appendix 3), muscles (Appendix 4), bones (Appendix 5), and peripheral nerve innervations of the upper and lower extremities (Appendices 6 and 7).

Appendices 8 through 12 describe areas that are relevant for the neuro exam, which is relevant in all of orthopedics and specifically applicable to spine. Nerve root assessments for upper and lower extremities are covered in Appendices 8 and 9. Dermatome distributions are depicted in Appendix 10. Reflexes, including deep tendon reflexes, upper motor neuron reflexes, and primitive reflexes, are covered in Appendix 11. The Muscle Strength Scale by the Medical Research Council is described in Appendix 12.

Appendices 13 through 18 are relevant for the practice of orthopedics on a daily basis, focusing on joint function and fracture management and classification. Normal ranges of motion are covered in Appendix 13. Aspirating joints for decompression or for fluid analysis and injecting joints for delivery of medication or dye are depicted and described in Appendix 14. Common fracture classifications throughout the body are described in Appendix 15. Traction pin placement for fracture management is described in Appendix 16. Finally, immobilization with casts, splints, and braces are described in Appendices 17 and 18.

Appendices 19 through 21 focus on specific medications that are pertinent to orthopedics, including analgesic medications (Appendix 19), prophylactic and therapeutic anticoagulation medications (Appendix 20), and antibiotics (Appendix 21).

The final appendices are a compendium of other important areas within orthopedics. Imaging in orthopedics, including modalities and radiographic views, are described in Appendix 22. Nerve conduction studies and electromyography, which are tests that are commonly used to assess nerve function, are covered in Appendix 23. Reading literature and understanding research in orthopedics is important to assess current findings that may change the practice of orthopedics (Appendix 24). Finally, Appendix 25 contains acronyms and names of national and international orthopedic associations.

Foreword

Dr. Antonia Chen is an orthopedic resident at the University of Pittsburgh Department of Orthopedic Surgery. After receiving her BS degree from Yale University and her MD degree from UMDNJ Robert Wood Johnson Medical School, Antonia joined our residency program in July 2008. Dr. Chen is an outstanding resident with a superior medical knowledge base and exceptional technical and clinical skills. In addition to her clinical knowledge, Dr. Chen is a prolific writer and has presented her scientific papers at local and national meetings. Here at the University of Pittsburgh, in a relatively short period of time, she has received 3 Pittsburgh Foundation grants, an OREF DePuy Resident Educational Grant, and a grant from the Scoliosis Research Society. In 2010, she was selected for the AAOS Clinician Scientist Development Program and is the first resident from our department to receive the Gold Foundation Humanism and Excellence in Teaching Award from the University of Pittsburgh Medical School Class of 2012. Dr. Chen has already established herself as one of our top residents and will undoubtedly become a leader in academic orthopedics.

In *Quick Reference Dictionary for Orthopedics*, you will find that Dr. Chen has compiled a comprehensive dictionary with 2235 orthopedic terms and unique appendices that highlight specific areas of orthopedics. This quick reference and user-friendly publication is geared for anyone that is exposed to the field of orthopedics, namely residents, medical students, nurses, therapists, trainers, medical secretaries, coders, and transcriptionists.

I extend my appreciation to Dr. Chen for undertaking this tremendous effort in assembling an everyday reference tool that provides a fast and easy way to access orthopedic terminology.

Freddie H. Fu, MD, DSc (Hon), DPs (Hon)
David Silver Professor and Chairman
Department of Orthopedic Surgery
University of Pittsburgh School of Medicine
Pittsburgh, Pennsylvania

A

A1 pulley: The most proximal annular pulley of the hand that originates from the volar plate of the metacarpal phalangeal joint. It is often the site where trigger finger occurs and may be surgically released to treat trigger finger.

abduction: Movement of a body part (usually the limbs) away from the midline of the body.

abduction bar: An orthopedic device used to position infant legs in abduction and external rotation. It is constructed by an aluminum bar with a pair of shoes fixed to the bar to position the feet (*see* Appendix 18). *Synonyms*: Denis Brown bar or brace, Fillauer bar, Tarso abduction bar.

abduction pillow: A triangle-shaped pillow placed between the legs to cause both legs to be abducted. Often used after total hip arthroplasty cases, especially from the posterior approach, to decrease the risk of dislocation in the immediate postoperative period.

abduction sling: A sling with an attached pillow to keep the arm in abduction. Often used for the postoperative immobilization of shoulder after a rotator cuff repair. Also known as a gunslinger brace (*see* Appendix 18).

abductor: A muscle that pulls a portion of the body away from the midline (memory hint: an abductor takes a person away).

abductor digiti minimi (ADM): A muscle that abducts the small finger or the little toe.

abductor hallucis (AH): A muscle that abducts the big toe. It originates from the calcaneal tuberosity and inserts in the proximal phalanx of the great toe.

abductor pollicis brevis (APB): A muscle that abducts the thumb. It originates from the scaphoid and trapezium and inserts in the lateral proximal phalanx of the thumb.

abductor pollicis longus (APL): A muscle that abducts and extends the thumb. It originates from the posterior radius/ulna and inserts in the base of the first metacarpal.

ablation: Removal of tissue, through surgery, chemotherapy, cryotherapy, or radiation. Term often used in orthopedic oncology.

above-knee amputation (AKA): An amputation above the level of the knee, often used in patients with severe peripheral vascular disease, trauma patients with no soft tissue coverage, or patients with infected knees (especially after total knee arthroplasty).

abrachia: A congenital anomaly characterized by the absence of arms.

abrasion: Loss of the epidermis or mucous membrane due to mechanical action, often due to a scraping injury.

abscess: A localized collection of pus within a cavity surrounded by soft tissue that is inflamed.

accessory navicular bone: A small secondary center of ossificiation in the tibialis posterior tendon next to the insertion on the navicular bone in the foot. May be surgically removed if too painful.

accuracy: A statistical term indicating that the experimental results agree with the accepted or true value of a test.

acetabuloplasty: A surgical procedure performed to remodel the hip socket to attempt to restore the anatomic shape. Used in the setting of acetabular dysplasia, various osteotomies (rotational, augmentation, capsular, or circumacetabular). May be performed to attempt to restore the natural shape of the acetabulum.

acetabulum/acetabular: The location where the femoral head articulates, or the hip socket. The normal anteversion of the acetabulum is 15 to 25 degrees, and the normal abduction of the acetabulum is 30 to 50 degrees.

acetylsalicylic acid (aspirin): A nonsteroidal anti-inflammatory drug that is used in orthopedics to reduce pain and inflammation; also used as a blood anticoagulant.

acheiria: A congenital anomaly in which one or both hands are missing.

Achilles tendon: Tendon connecting the triceps surae to the calcaneus composed of the tendons of the gastrocnemius and soleus muscles. This muscle is often lengthened or released in pediatric patients with clubfeet and is often ruptured in middle-aged males while playing sports. *Synonyms:* Tendoachilles, heel cord.

achondroplasia: A congenital anomaly resulting in shortened limbs due to slowed growth in the ossification centers of cartilage in the long bones. May be inherited from parents with achondroplasia or may be due to a genetic mutation in the fibroblast growth factor receptor 3 (FGFR 3) gene on chromosome 4.

aclasia: Condition in which abnormal tissue is derived from and is continuous with normal tissues.

acquired disorders/deformities: Diseases, deformities, or dysfunctions that are not genetic but produced by influences originating outside of the organism.

acromegaly: Increased secretion of growth hormone from the pituitary gland that results in excessive enlargement of bone in the extremities, hands, feet, and head.

acromioplasty: Surgical procedure by which the antero-inferior portion of the acromion is removed, as the acromion mechanically compresses the rotator cuff during shoulder movement. This may be done either arthroscopically or through an open approach.

acromium: A lateral projection of bone from the scapula that forms the superior border of the shoulder girdle.

active assisted range of motion (AAROM): Amount of motion at a given joint achieved by a person using his or her own muscle strength with assistance.

active range of motion (AROM): Amount of motion at a given joint achieved by a person using his or her own muscle strength.

activities of daily living (ADL): Activities required for independence in everyday living, including self-care, communication, and mobility (eg, transfers, ambulation, dressing, grooming, bathing, eating, and using the toilet).

acupressure: Use of touch at specific points along the meridians of the body to release the tensions that cause various physical symptoms.

acupuncture: Use of needles at specific points along the meridians of the body to release energy or to induce anesthesia. Developed by the Ancient Chinese and may sometimes be used as an adjunct to treatment or prevention of diseases.

acute: A sudden onset of a condition of short and intense duration. *Antonym*: Chronic.

acute respiratory distress syndrome (ARDS): A life-threatening lung condition that prevents enough oxygen from getting into the blood. May occur postoperatively and present with respiratory distress.

adactyly: Congenital anomaly in which there are no fingers or toes.

adamantinoma: A very rare and slow-growing tumor that often arises in the tibia or jaw. *Synonym*: Ameloblastoma.

adaptive equipment: A variety of equipment used to aid patients in performing movements, tasks, or activities (eg, raised toilet seats and hospital beds).

adduction: Movement toward the midline of the body.

adductor: A muscle that pulls a portion of the body toward the midline.

adductor brevis: A muscle that adducts the thigh. It originates from the body of the inferior pubic ramus and inserts on the pectineal line, or the upper portion of the linea aspera.

adductor hallucis: A muscle that adducts the big toe. It originates from the metatarsals and inserts on the proximal phalanx of the great toe.

adductor longus: A muscle that adducts the thigh. It originates from the body of the inferior pubis and inserts on the middle third of the linea aspera.

adductor magnus: A muscle that adducts the thigh as well as flexes and extends the thigh. It originates from the ischiopubic ramus and ischial tuberosity and inserts in the linea aspera (adductor tubercle).

adductor pollicis (ADP): A muscle that adducts the thumb. It originates from the capitate, second and third metacarpals, and inserts in the base of the proximal phalanx of the thumb.

adhesion: Soft tissue scarring that forms fibrotic tissue resulting from injury, inflammation, or previous surgery.

adhesive capsulitis: Inflammation of the joint capsule that causes limitation of mobility or immobility of the joint. Often occurs in the shoulder and results in frozen shoulder.

adolescent idiopathic scoliosis (AIS): A curvature of the spine that has an onset around the beginning of puberty or before skeletal maturity. There is no known cause.

Adson forceps: A type of nonlocking forceps with a short handle and 2 teeth on the end that locks with 1 tooth on the opposite side. May also be called pick-ups.

advance directives: Living wills and care instruction in which a competent adult expresses his or her wishes regarding medical management in the event of a serious illness.

Advanced Trauma Life Support (ATLS): A systematic and concise approach to the early care of trauma patients.

advancement flap: A surgical technique by which a flap of skin is advanced from an adjacent area to cover another area. Often used to cover amputated fingertips.

aerobe: A microorganism that lives and grows in the presence of oxygen.

alcoholism: A chronic disease characterized by an uncontrollable urge to consume alcoholic beverages excessively. These patients are at risk for many complications, including withdrawing from alcohol, which may lead to a metabolic disease called delirium tremens.

allele: Alternative form of a gene coded for a particular trait.

Allman classification: A fracture classification system for clavicle fractures (*see* Appendix 15).

allograft: Transplantation of a biological sample obtained from another source of the same species (eg, bone graft taken from a cadaver).

alopecia: Absence or loss of hair; baldness.

alpha error: When the null hypothesis is rejected, the probability of being wrong or the probability of rejecting it when it should have been accepted. *Synonym*: Type I error.

alpha-fetoprotein (AFP): A protein produced by the fetus that can be found in the amniotic fluid in utero and in the bloodstream of the mother. May be elevated in patients with open neural tube defects, such as spina bifida, Down syndrome, and cancer.

ALPSA (anterior labral periosteal sleeve avulsion) lesion: An avulsion of the anterior labrum with a concomitant periosteal sleeve that is associated with shoulder dislocations.

ambulate: To walk.

ambulatory care: Care delivered on an outpatient basis.

ambulatory surgery center (ASC): A surgery center where surgical procedures are performed on an outpatient basis.

amelia: Congenital anomaly characterized by the absence of extremities.

amenorrhea: Absence of a monthly menstruation that may result in decreased bone density. May be due to pregnancy, birth control medication, anorexia, endocrine disease, hormonal imbalances, or stress.

amniotic band: A band of amniotic membrane that may constrict a fetus' extremities while in utero that may result in loss of part or all of a limb.

amphiarthrotic joint: A synarthrosis by which 2 bones are connected by fibrocartilage (symphysis) or an interosseous ligament (syndesmosis). Examples include vertebral body articulations within the spine and tibiofibular articulations. *Synonym*: Amphiarthrosis.

amplitude: The maximal height of a waveform, either from the baseline or peak to peak.

amputation: Partial or complete removal of a limb; may be congenital or acquired (traumatic or surgical).

amyloid: An insoluble fibrous protein polysaccharide.

amyloidosis: Disease in which amyloid is deposited in organs (eg, kidney, gastrointestinal tract, lungs, and skin); associated with conditions such as multiple myeloma.

amyotonia: Lack of muscle tone; may be congenital or acquired.

amyotrophic lateral sclerosis (ALS): A disease characterized by progressive degeneration of spinal cord nerves that control voluntary motor function. This leads to muscle weakness and decreased function, first in the extremities and later in the chest wall. *Synonyms*: Lou Gehrig disease, motor neuron disease.

amyotrophy: Muscular atrophy or wasting away.

anaerobe: A microorganism that grows in the absence of oxygen.

analgesia: Absence of pain sensitivity; patients may experience the stimulus (pressure) but it is not noxious.

analgesic: Drug for reducing pain.

analysis: An examination of the nature of something for the purpose of prediction or comparison.

analysis of covariance (ANCOVA): A statistical test used to control and eliminate the effects of a specified variable known to correlate with the dependent variable.

analysis of variance (ANOVA, F ratio): A statistical test used to establish whether a significant difference exists among the means of multiple continuous variables.

anaphylactic shock: A condition due to an allergic reaction where vasodilation occurs and blood circulation is inadequate. It is also associated with severe bronchoconstriction to the point where the individual is unable to breathe.

anconeus: A muscle that extends the forearm. It originates from the lateral epicondyle of the humerus and inserts in the proximal ulna.

anemia: A condition in which there is a reduction in the number or volume of red blood cells, as measured by hemoglobin or hematocrit. Postoperative orthopedic patients may experience this and may present with hypotension, tachycardia, paleness, dizziness, and syncopal episodes.

anesthesia: Absence of sensibility to stimuli with or without loss of consciousness.

anesthetic: Drug that reduces or eliminates sensation. It can affect the whole body (eg, nitrous oxide, a general anesthetic) or a particular part of the body (eg, Xylocaine, a local anesthetic).

aneurysmal bone cyst (ABC): Benign osteolytic tumor of the bone that is defined by blood-filled spaces within the bone separated by fibrous septae.

angiography: Injection of a contrast so that the blood vessels can be visualized using imaging, like x-ray, computed tomography (CT), and magnetic resonance imaging (MRI). Often done after knee dislocations.

angiolipoma: Benign tumor containing fat and small blood vessels.

angioma: Benign tumors composed of blood vessels.

angiomatosis of bone: Angiomas within bone.

angiomyolipoma: Benign tumor containing muscle, fat, and small blood vessels.

angioneurotic edema: Edema of an extremity due to any neurosis primarily affecting the blood vessels resulting from a disorder of the vasomotor system, such as angiospasm, angioparesis, or angioparalysis.

angulation deformity: An abnormal bend within a structure. In orthopedics, often refers to a fracture in the long bone resulting in nonanatomic alignment.

anisomelia: A congenital defect in which there is a limb length discrepancy at birth.

Ankle Brachial Index (ABI): An objective measurement of blood flow calculated by the systolic blood pressure in the leg divided by the systolic blood pressure in the arm. These are often done with Doppler ultrasound. An ABI < 0.9 is often indicative of peripheral vascular disease, and an ABI > 1.2 is often due to calcified vessels.

ankle–foot orthosis (AFO): An external device that controls the foot and ankle and can facilitate knee positioning and muscle response (*see* Appendix 18).

ankylosing spondylitis (AS): An autoimmune disorder in which the connective tissue between the vertebrae and sacroiliac joints becomes inflamed and fuses. Spine motion is severely limited and these patients are at increased risk of spine fractures. Special care must be taken when positioning these patients to ensure that there is no neck hyperextension.

ankylosis: Condition of the joints in which they become stiffened and nonfunctional. Abnormal immobility and consolidation of a joint due to surgery or disease.

annular: Ring shaped. May refer to a ligament, band of tissue, or fibrotic tissue comprising a portion of the vertebral disc.

annular pulley in the hand: Circular fibrous sheaths that attach to the joint capsules and shafts of the phalanges in the hand. Labeled A1 through A5 from proximal to distal.

anomaly: Deviation from the norm.

anoxia: Absence or deficiency of oxygen in the issues. May lead to tissue death.

antalgic: A compensatory behavior attempting to avoid or lessen pain, usually applied to gait or movement.

antebrachium: The distal portion of the arm between the wrist and the elbow that contains the radius and ulna. *Synonym*: Forearm.

antecubital: Anterior portion of the elbow.

anterior: Toward the front of the body. *Synonym*: Ventral.

anterior cord syndrome: Trauma or ischemia to the anterior portion of the spinal cord resulting in paralysis with intact sensation.

anterior cruciate ligament (ACL): Ligament that connects the femur to the tibia and prevents anterior translation and rotation of the tibia relative to the femur. Often injured or ruptured in athletes who perform cutting maneuvers.

anterior drawer test: A physical exam maneuver where the knee is flexed to 90 degrees and the tibia is pulled forward. Excessive anterior translation indicates that the anterior cruciate ligament (ACL) is injured.

anterior horn cell: Motor neuron located anteriorly in the spinal cord that is similar in shape to a pointed projection, such as the paired processes on the head of various animals.

anterior inferior iliac spine (AIIS): The lower front point on the iliac wing of the pelvis where the rectus femoris muscle attaches.

anterior longitudinal ligament (ALL): A strong connective tissue band that connects vertebral bodies in the front.

anterior superior iliac spine (ASIS): The higher front portion of the iliac wing of the pelvis where the sartorius muscle attaches.

anterolateral: An anatomic location toward the front and away from the midline.

anteromedial: An anatomic location toward the front and toward the midline.

anteroposterior (AP): A radiographic projection where the x-ray beam passes from the front (anterior) to the back (posterior).

anterotalofibular ligament (ATFL): A fibrous connective tissue attached from the anterior distal fibula to the talus that prevents anterior translation of the foot. It is the most commonly injured ligament in lateral ankle sprains.

anteversion: An anatomic position term that describes a structure that is rotated forward, or toward, the front of the body. Often used to describe the femur or acetabulum. *Antonym*: Retroversion.

antibiotic: Chemical substance that has the ability to inhibit or kill bacteria in the body.

antibody: A protein belonging to a class of proteins called immunoglobulins. A molecule produced by the immune system of the body in response to a specific antigen to combat infectious agents.

anticoagulant: A substance that prevents or slows blood clotting. Often used after orthopedic procedures to prevent deep vein thrombosis and pulmonary emboli.

antigen: A substance foreign to the body that stimulates the formation or release of antibodies.

anti-inflammatory drug: Any pharmacologic agent that reduces inflammation but does not eliminate the causing agent. This group of medications includes steroids and cyclooxygenase (COX) inhibitors.

antineoplastic agents: Substances, procedures, or measures used to treat cancer, administered with the purposes of destroying or inhibiting the production of malignant cells.

antinuclear antibody (ANA): A protein within the host's own immune system that reacts with the cell nucleus. Often elevated in patients with rheumatoid arthritis, systemic lupus erythematosus, or other autoimmune or connective tissue diseases.

antioxidant: A substance that scavenges free radicals and prevents cellular damage to slow the oxidation of hydrocarbon, oils, and fats.

anuria: Absence of urine excretion. May present as a postoperative complication due to hypovolemia, obstruction, or a physiological disorder.

AO (Arbeitsgemeinschaft für Osteosynthesefragen): An organization formed by Swiss orthopedic surgeons in 1958 that established the use of plates and screws for bone fixation. Also known as the Association for the Study of Internal Fixation (ASIF; *see* Appendix 15).

AO fracture classification: A fracture classification scheme developed by the AO based on an alphanumeric system. The first 2 numbers describe the location of the fracture, and the following letter and 2 numbers describe the morphological characteristic of the fracture (*see* Appendix 15).

AO technique: Four principles to fracture fixation developed by the AO foundation, which include anatomic reduction, stable fixation, soft tissue preservation, and early mobilization.

Apert syndrome: Congenital abnormality due to mutations in the fibroblast growth factor receptor 2 (FGFR 2) gene that results in a flat forehead, depressed nose, skull malformation, and fused fingers and toes. *Synonyms*: Acrocephalosyndactyly, acrocephalosyndactylia.

aplasia: A congenital anomaly in which there is incomplete or no development of an organ or tissue. May be seen in the odontoid.

Apley grind test: A physical exam test for meniscal tears where the patient is placed prone, the knee is flexed to 90 degrees, and a downward and external rotation force is placed on the knee to see whether pain is produced.

apnea: Temporary cessation of breathing. Often associated with obese patients who experience apnea episodes when sleeping. These patients may require continuous pulse oximeter monitoring, especially in the postoperative period.

aponeurosis: Fibrous or membraneous tendon-like tissue that connects a muscle to the part that the muscle moves.

aponeurotic fibroma: A benign calcifying tumor found within the aponeuroses of the hands and feet of children or adolescents that presents as a painless nodule.

apophysis: An outgrowth from bone that contains the center of ossification that is not adjacent to a joint. Examples include the iliac crest and the greater trochanter of the femur.

apophysitis: Inflammation of the apophysis.

apoptosis: Programmed cell death.

appendicular: The upper and lower extremities.

approximation: Bringing the cutaneous edges of a surgical or traumatic wound together with sutures.

arachnodactyly: Fingers that are elongated, often seen in connective tissue disorders like Marfan syndrome.

arcuate: Anatomic description for being shaped like a bow or arc.

Arizona brace: (Arizona AFO, Mesa, Arizona) A trademark lace-up ankle brace used to restrict motion at the ankle (*see* Appendix 18).

Arnold Chiari malformation: A disease process in which the cerebellum is displaced inferiorly through the foramen magnum that causes hydrocephalus from an outflow obstruction. Type I is the most common, in which there is herniation of the cerebellar tonsils that may clinically manifest with headaches. Type II has greater cerebellar displacement and is commonly associated with lumbar myelomeningocele, which may lead to paralysis.

arterial insufficiency: Inadequate blood supply in the arterial system usually caused by stenosis or occlusion proximal to the inadequately supplied area.

arterial thrombosis: Obstruction of an arterial blood vessel formed by the coagulation and fibrosis of blood at a particular site.

arteriosclerosis: Thickening, hardening, and a loss of elasticity of the walls of the arteries.

arteriovenous malformation (AVM): Direct connection between arteries and veins that skips capillaries and appears as a configuration of twisted blood vessels.

arthralgia: Pain within a joint. *Synonym*: Arthrodynia.

arthritis: Inflammation of the joints that may be chronic or acute. May be degenerative, autoimmune, or due to infection.

arthrocentesis: Entering a joint capsule with a needle to aspirate or inject fluid.

arthrodesis: Surgical procedure of fusing a joint. Requires removal of cartilage to allow bony apposition followed by surgical fixation to make the joint rigid. *Synonym*: Fusion.

arthrofibrosis: Excessive scar tissue formation within a joint that limits motion.

arthrogram: Injection of dye or air into a joint cavity to better image the joint, specifically looking for soft tissue defects. Also known as an arthrography (*see* Appendix 22).

arthrogryposis (arthrogryposis multiplex congenita, AMC): A congenital condition characterized by multiple joint contractures that often leads to muscle weakness.

arthroplasty: Surgical reconstruction of a joint.

arthroscopy: Surgical procedure in which a small camera is inserted into a joint for visualization though a small portal. Most often performed in knees and shoulders but also used for hips, ankles, wrists, and elbows.

arthrotomy: Surgical incision of a joint.

articular cartilage: A smooth white tissue composed of hyaline that covers the articulating surface of bones. The loss of articular cartilage is osteoarthritis.

articulation: The juncture between 2 or more bones.

artifact: An artificial or extraneous feature introduced into an observation that may stimulate a relevant feature of that observation.

aseptic: Free from infection or septic material; sterile.

asphyxia: Condition of insufficient oxygen.

aspirate: (1) To remove fluid from a joint or body cavity. (2) To inhale vomitus, mucus, or food into the respiratory tract. Surgical patients do not eat the night before surgery because eating causes a postoperative anesthesia complication worsened by nausea.

assessment: Process by which data are gathered, hypotheses formulated, and decisions made for further action. To be included prior to developing a plan for patients.

assistive devices: A variety of implements or equipment used to aid patients in performing tasks or movements, which include crutches, canes, walkers, wheelchairs, power devices, and braces.

assistive living facility: A living situation in which persons live in community housing with attendant care that offers housing, meals, and personal care, plus extras such as housekeeping, transportation, and recreation.

asymmetric: Having an inequality or unequal parts, often used in orthopedics to describe extremities.

asynergy: Lack of coordination between muscle groups that results in gait or motion abnormality, often seen in cerebral palsy patients.

ataxia: Poor balance and awkward movement. One disorder seen in the orthopedic patient population is Friedreich ataxia.

athletic pubalgia: Groin pain that affects athletes due to dilation of the superficial ring of the inguinal canal. Also known as sports hernia or sportsman's hernia.

atlanto-axial: The region between the atlas (C1) and axis (C2) that often subluxes in patients with rheumatoid arthritis or Down syndrome.

atlas: The first cervical vertebrae (C1) that supports the skull.

atonic: Having a loss of muscle tone.

atrophy: The decrease in size of a normally developed organ or tissue due to lack of use or deficient nutrition or vascular supply. Often seen in muscles after wearing a cast.

attenuation: Stretching or thinning of tendons and other connective tissue so that they become weak and face the possibility of rupture.

autograft: Transplantation of a biological sample obtained from the host source (eg, skin graft taken from the patient's own body).

autoimmunity: Condition in which the body has developed a sensitivity to some of its own tissues.

autologous: Obtained from oneself. May refer to blood or a graft.

autolysis: Disintegration or liquefaction of tissue or cells by the body's own mechanisms.

autonomic nervous system (ANS): The portion of the nervous system not under voluntary control, consisting of the sympathetic and parasympathetic nervous systems.

autosomal dominant: Genetic trait carried on the autosome that prevails over other traits. Examples of conditions that are often autosomal dominant and are pertinent to orthopedics include Ehlers-Danlos, Marfan, achondroplasia, and neurofibromatosis.

autosomal recessive: Genetic trait carried on the autosome that is expressed only if both parents have the autosome. Examples of conditions that are often autosomal recessive and are pertinent to orthopedics include Gaucher disease and Friedreich ataxia.

autosome: Any chromosome other than the X and Y (sex chromosomes). In humans, there are 22 pairs of autosomes.

avascular: Tissue without a blood supply. May be physiologic (cartilage) or pathologic (skin or bone).

avascular necrosis (AVN): Lack of blood supply to the bone, often leading to bone collapse and destruction. Most common in the hips and shoulders. Causes include high-dose steroids and alcoholism.

avulsion: Tearing away of a ligament or tendon from its attachment or fracturing a bone fragment from the main bone.

axial skeleton: Bones that form the longitudinal axis of the body; consists of the skull, vertebral column, thorax, and sternum.

axilla: Area located inferior to the humerus and glenohumeral joint. The brachial plexus passes through the inferior portion of the axilla.

axillary lateral view: A technique to capture radiographs of the glenohumeral joint to ensure that the shoulder is located. The patient is supine on the table and the arm is abducted to 90 degrees. The x-ray cassette is placed superior to the shoulder and the beam is parallel to the body and directed toward the midline of the body.

axis: (1) A line, real or imaginary, that runs through the center of the body. Anatomical directions are defined by this line, such as medial (close to the midline) and lateral (away from the midline). (2) The second cervical vertebrae (C2) around which the atlas (C1) rotates.

axon: Long part of a nerve cell that sends information away from the cell, across a synapse, to the dendrites of another cell.

axonotmesis: A more severe form of damage to a nerve, where the axon is interrupted with subsequent wallerian degeneration; connective tissues of the nerve including the Schwann cells, epineurium, endoneurium, and perineurium remain intact.

azotema: Presence of nitrogenous bodies, especially urea, in the blood.

B

Babinski reflex: Extension of the great toe when the plantar surface of the foot is stroked from the heel to the toes. It is physiologically normal in infants up until the age of one, but it is a sign of upper motor neuron disease in adults.

bacitracin: A topical antibacterial ointment used on wounds.

bactericidal: An agent that is capable of killing bacteria. An example of a bacteriostatic surgical preparation option is iodopovidone, and an example of bactericidal antibiotics is the class of beta-lactam antibiotics.

bacteriostatic: An agent that is capable of inhibiting the growth or multiplication of bacteria but is unable to kill it. An example of a bacteriostatic surgical preparation option is alcohol, and an example of bacteriostatic antibiotics is the class of macrolides.

Bado classification: A fracture classification system for Monteggia fractures based on the dislocation of the radial head (*see* Appendix 15).

Baker cyst: A collection of fluid within a sac in the popliteal fossa (posterior knee) filled with synovial fluid from the knee. Often seen in patients with osteoarthritis. *Synonym*: Popliteal cyst.

balanced hemivertebrae: A congenital anomaly in which the vertebral column is composed of 2 half-vertebrae that are balanced mirror images of each other so the overall spine alignment is preserved.

bamboo spine: A spine that looks like bamboo on x-ray, which is advanced stage of ankylosing spondylitis.

bandage: A soft dressing that covers a wound or applies compression to a region of the body.

Bankart lesion: An injury to the anterior–inferior glenoid labrum as a result of traumatic anterior shoulder dislocation.

Barlow test: A physical exam to determine whether a neonate has dislocated hips due to developmental dysplasia of the hip. The hips are flexed, the legs are adducted, and a posterior force is applied to attempt to dislocate the hips.

Barton wrist fracture: Fracture of the distal radius with concomitant dislocation of the distal radioulnar joint.

baseline: The known value or quantity representing the normal/reference background level against which a response to intervention can be measured. Example: Muscle strength testing; subjective levels can be compared on a daily basis (*see* Appendix 12).

basilar: The base of a structure. For example, a basicervical femoral neck fracture occurs at the base of femoral neck.

Baumann angle: The angle between the humeral shaft and the physis of the capitellum (lateral condyle of the humerus) used to determine the alignment of supracondylar humerus fractures. A normal Baumann angle ranges from 75 to 85 degrees. *Synonym*: Humeral capitellar angle.

bayonet apposition: When the fractured ends of long bone have contact on one cortex so that the fracture heals in a side-by-side position. The name derives from the appearance of a bayonet attached to a rifle.

beach chair position: The surgical positioning of a patient for shoulder surgery with the patient flexed approximately 60 to 70 degrees at the hips and reclined with the knees flexed.

bean bag: A device used in the operating room to assist with positioning the patient. It is a pellet-filled bag that becomes rigid when air is removed through suction, allowing for customized positioning of the patient.

Becker muscular dystrophy: A genetic condition characterized by weakness of the lower extremities that is milder than Duchenne muscular dystrophy.

Beck syndrome: A condition in which the anterior spinal artery is occluded, resulting in motor impairment without sensory changes. *Synonym*: Anterior spinal artery syndrome.

below-knee amputation (BKA): Removal of the leg below the knee joint. Commonly performed for patients with severe ischemic changes, severe infections, or irreparable trauma to the lower leg.

bends (decompression sickness, diver disease): A rapid decrease in pressure that causes nitrogen bubble formation in blood and results in soft tissue and bone damage. Patients often present with joint pain (most often the shoulder), low back pain due to bubbles within the spine, and/or skin lesions. Patients are treated in a hyperbaric chamber.

beneficence: The medically ethical act of doing good for the benefit of the patient. One part of the Hippocratic Oath.

benign: Not dangerous to one's health or life.

benign myotonia congenital: A congenital disorder characterized by decreased muscle tone and weakness that often spontaneously resolves. *Synonyms:* Floppy baby syndrome, Oppenheim syndrome.

Bennett fracture: A 2-part intra-articular fracture at the base of the thumb metacarpal bone.

beta error: When the null hypothesis is accepted, the probability of being wrong or the probability of accepting it when it should have been rejected. *Synonym:* Type 2 error.

biceps: A large muscle with 2 heads of origin. May be found in the upper extremity (biceps brachii) and in the lower extremity (biceps femoris).

biceps brachii: A muscle that flexes the elbow. The long head originates from the supraglenoid tubercle and the short head originates from the coracoid process. They both insert into the radial tuberosity in the proximal radius.

biceps femoris: A hamstring muscle that extends the thigh and flexes the knee. The long head originates from the ischial tuberosity and the short head originates from the linea aspera. Both insert into the head of the fibula by a common tendon.

bicipital: (1) Muscle origin having 2 heads (eg, rectus femoris muscle). (2) Related to the biceps muscle.

Bïer block: Regional anesthesia performed by injecting an anesthetic into a vein that has been exsanguinated by a tourniquet. The location of the injection is distal to the tourniquet. Often performed in the upper extremity.

bifurcation: The site of division into 2 branches, as in an artery. Often the area of atherosclerotic deposits.

bilateral: Pertaining to or affecting both sides of the body.

bimalleolar fracture: A distal fracture of both the tibia and the fibula, often of the lateral and medial malleoli.

biocompatible: Materials that do not harm tissue and do not cause immune rejection.

bioethics: Application of ethics to health care.

biofilm: An aggregation of bacteria that forms a solid substrate that adheres to surfaces. These bacteria, such as *Staphylococcus aureus*, have an affinity for metal surfaces and make eradication of infection more difficult from orthopedic implants.

biomaterial: Material that is biologically compatible with the host and may be implanted.

biomechanics: Study of anatomy, physiology, and physics as applied to the human body.

biopsy: Removal of a portion of tissue or fluid for pathological and/or laboratory analysis. Varying degrees of invasiveness, ranging from a needle biopsy to an open biopsy.

bipartite: Composed of 2 parts (eg, congenital anomaly of the patella resulting in a bipartite patella). *Synonym*: Bifid.

bipolar hemiarthroplasty: A proximal femoral prosthesis with 2 articulations, one between the neck and head and another between the head and the cup (acetabulum for hip). In the hip, it is a prosthesis used to treat displaced femoral neck fractures.

Birbeck granule: A structure within immature dendritic cells of the epidermis (Langerhans cells) that is racket-shaped and membrane bound. *Synonym*: Langerhans granule.

bivalve: To split a cast into 2 parts to allow for swelling.

blanching: Becoming white with pressure; maximum pallor.

blastoma: A tumor composed of immature and undifferentiated cells (eg, chondroblastoma; a tumor consisting of undifferentiated cartilage cells).

block: A regional injection of an anesthetic agent to block nerve function to a body part.

blood: Fluid that supplies oxygen, nutrients, and a vehicle to remove waste from the tissues in the body. Blood is composed of red blood cells, white blood cells, platelets, and plasma.

bloodborne pathogen: Infectious disease spread by contact with blood; for example, acquired immune deficiency syndrome (AIDS) and hepatitis B and C.

blood pressure (BP): Pressure of the blood against the walls of the blood vessels. A normal blood pressure as defined by the American Heart Association is less than 120 mm Hg during systole and less than 80 mm Hg during diastole.

blood urea nitrogen (BUN): The serum measurement of the waste product urea nitrogen from protein breakdown that is normally filtered by the kidneys. The BUN is elevated in renal failure (greater than 20 mg/dL).

Blount disease: A growth arrest of the proximal medial physeal growth plate in the tibia resulting in varus aligment (bowlegged).

Blumensaat line: A line in the condylar femoral notch located along the posterior slope. Visualized on a lateral radiograph of the knee and used to determine the relative position of the patella.

blunt dissection: The separation of soft tissues with a finger or blunted instrument.

bone: Dense connective tissue that provides structural support in the form of the skeleton. Composed of carbonated hydroxyapatite and type I collagen. New forming bone is called woven bone. Types of bone include cancellous, cortical, flat, irregular, and sesamoid bones.

bone age: The age of a child based on radiographs of the hand and wrist assessing the degree of skeletal maturity. Often determined using the Greulich-Pyle atlas. May not correlate to chronological age.

bone bank: The location where bone from live donors or cadavers is stored.

bone cyst: A cavity within a bone that may be empty or fluid filled and is often benign.

bone density: The amount of bone mineralization in the skeleton. This is typically quantified using a dual-emission x-ray absorptiometry (DEXA) scan and reported as a T score or Z score.

bone dysostosis: Defective bone formation.

bone graft: Transplantation of bone either from the patient (autograft) or another source (allograft/xenograft). Often used to fill defects or stimulate bone growth.

bone island: An area of dense bone seen on x-ray due to an increase in calcium deposits.

bone lacuna: A small cavity in the bone matrix that contains an osteocyte that connects to other lacunas with canaliculi.

bone marrow: Spongy tissue that fills the porous medullary canal in the diaphysis of bones composed of blood forming agents when young and increased fat when adult.

bone matrix: An interlocking framework mostly composed of collagen and carbonated hydroxyapatite that gives bone its structure and relative flexibility.

bone morphogenic protein (BMP): A growth factor that stimulates bone and cartilage formation. Though there are many different BMPs, only BMP 2 and 7 are commercially used to stimulate bone growth in tibial fractures and in spine fusions.

bone putty: A paste composed of demineralized bone and a carrier that conforms to the area it is filling. This bone graft can fill a defect and is eventually replaced by natural bone.

bone remodeling: The cyclic process of bone formation and breakdown that regulates the repair, maintenance, and growth of bone.

bone scan: A nuclear imaging study that injects a radioactive marker that collects in bone. Detects areas of increased activity in bone and may be used to diagnose tumors, infection, implant loosening or fractures (*see* Appendix 22).

bone skid: A surgical instrument used to slide a bone in and out of a socket. This instrument can be used, for example, to slide the femoral head out of the acetabulum.

bone stimulator: A device that utilizes electromagnetic fields or ultrasound to increase healing in fractured bones. Controversial usefulness in fracture nonunions.

bone wax: A substance composed of oil, wax, and antiseptic agents that is used to stop bleeding from bone.

bony mallet: A fracture of the distal phalanx that results in an extensor tendon avulsion that presents with a flexed distal interphalangeal joint. Also known as a mallet fracture.

bossing: A localized protuberance or swelling.

Boston brace: A molded chest and back brace used to control thoracic and lumbar scoliosis (*see* Appendix 18).

boutonnière deformity: Abnormality of the hand that causes metacarpal phalangeal joint hyperextension and interphalangeal joint flexion. Often caused by trauma (rupture of the central slip) or rheumatoid arthritis.

bovie: An electrocautery device used to cauterize bleeding vessels.

bowlegs: Varus deformity of the lower extremities.

bowler thumb: Ulnar digital nerve irritation of the thumb due to thumb compression within the holes of a bowling ball.

boxer fracture: A transverse fracture of the fifth metacarpal of the hand, often after delivering a punching blow.

brace: A device used to correct a position, provide support, and/or immobilize a body part in order to restore function. Also known as an orthosis (*see* Appendix 18).

brachialis: A muscle that flexes the forearm that originates from the distal anterior humerus and inserts in the ulnar tuberosity.

brachial plexus: Network of nerves that originate at the C5, C6, C7, C8, and T1 nerve roots and innervates the upper extremity. Divided into 5 sections: roots, trunks, divisions, cords, and branches.

brachioradialis: A muscle that flexes the forearm. It originates from the lateral supracondylar humerus and inserts in the lateral distal radius.

bradycardia: A slow heartbeat (less than 60 beats/minute). May be physiologically normal for some individuals, mostly athletes.

breast stroker's knee: Medial collateral ligament (MCL) strain in swimmers due to the whipping kick used in breast stroke.

bridging technique: A surgical technique of fracture fixation where the fracture is spanned by hardware and the fracture heals by secondary intention.

Brodie's abscess: A localized bone infection that is walled off by the body in an attempt to heal it.

Bröstrom procedure: A surgical procedure performed in the foot to repair the lateral ligaments (anterior talofibular ligament, calcaneofibular ligament) and tightening of the extensor retinaculum to correct ankle instability.

Brown-Séquard syndrome: Incomplete spinal cord injury affecting half of the spinal cord that results in motor loss on one side of the body and pain and temperature sensory loss on the contralateral side.

brown tumor: A mass of fibrous tissue composed of hemosiderin found in the bones of hyperparathyroidism patients.

Brudzinski's reflex: A sign of meningitis that results in leg pain when the neck is passively flexed.

bruit: An abnormal sound due to turbulent blood flow in a blood vessel or the heart.

bucket handle meniscal tear: A type of laceration in the central meniscus where both edges of the meniscus are still fixed.

buckle fracture: A break in the bone that does not fully disrupt both cortices; occurs in the pediatric population. *Synonym*: Torus fracture.

Buck traction: Skin traction of the lower leg by applying a boot and adding weights. Often used in elderly patients with hip fractures.

bulbocavernosus reflex: A physical exam method used to determine the end of spinal shock in spinal cord injury by squeezing the end of the penis to see whether the rectal sphincter spontaneously contracts. In females, this maneuver may be performed by inserting a foley and tugging on the end of the foley to see whether the rectum spontaneously contracts.

bunion: An enlargement of the first metatarsophalangeal joint at the head of the first metatarsal resulting in the first toe (hallux) deviating laterally (valgus) from the midline. *Synonym*: Hallux valgus.

bunionectomy: The removal of a bunion.

burner: An injury due to contact sports (often football) with a stretch or compression force across the brachial plexus that results in sudden pain and tingling from the neck and through the arms and fingers. *Synonym*: Stinger.

burr: An instrument used to shave bone.

bursa: A sac that contains synovial fluid. Bursas are located in superficial fascia in areas where movement takes place and aid in decreasing friction. Locations include the subacromial space, olecranon, hip (greater trochanter), and knee.

bursitis: Inflammation of a bursa resulting from injury, infection, or rheumatoid synovitis.

burst fracture: A break in the vertebrae involving the anterior and middle columns, leaving the posterior column intact. Severity is determined by the amount of neurologic deficit, the loss of vertebral body height, the amount of canal compromise, and the severity of bony deformity.

butterfly fragment: A triangular piece of bone splintered from the main fracture; resembles a butterfly with outstretched wings.

buttonhole: To create a hole or rent in the skin that is not physiologic. A bone fracture fragment may poke through the skin, or a subcutaneous suture may accidentally pierce the skin.

buttress plate: A surgical piece of hardware that supports the bone to prevent a fracture fragment from sliding into the bone.

bypass: A surgically created detour between 2 points in a physiological pathway to circumvent obstructions. An example is a vascular bypass created to supply blood flow to an extremity after damage to the popliteal artery due to a knee dislocation.

cable plate: Surgical hardware designed to attach to the bones with cables that encircle bone. Often used for fracture fixation where screws are not an option, especially after shoulder and hip arthroplasty where an implant fills the canal.

cadaver: A corpse often used for dissection.

café au lait spots: Light brown pigmentation of skin, from the French "coffee with milk." Associated with various diseases, including neurofibromatosis and fibrous dysplasia.

calcaneocavus deformity: A deformity with a dorsiflexed heel and plantarflexed forefoot that results in a high arch, often seen in cerebral palsy patients. *Synonym*: Talipes calcaneocavus.

calcaneocuboid joint: An articulation between the calcaneus and the cuboid that provides stability to the lateral foot. They are connected by 5 ligaments: the articular capsular, plantar calcaneocuboid, dorsal calcaneocuboid, long plantar, and bifurcated ligaments.

calcaneovalgus deformity: A flexible flatfoot deformity where the foot is abducted, often seen in infants due to fetal malpositioning. *Synonym*: Talipes calcaneovalgus.

calcaneovarus deformity: A deformity that combines talipes varus and talipes calcaneus, which results in a foot that is dorsiflexed, inverted, and adducted. *Synonym*: Talipes calcaneovarus.

calcaneus: The bone of the heel. *Synonym*: Os calcis.

calcar: A dense area of bone, including a spur or osteophyte. Often describing the dense shelf of bone on the medial portion of the femoral neck.

calcification: The deposit of calcium salts. It is physiological in tissue such as bone and teeth but is pathological in soft tissue.

Chen AF, ed.
Quick Reference Dictionary for Orthopedics (pp 26-43).

calcific tendonitis: Deposits of hydroxyapatite in tendons. Most commonly seen in the supraspinatus (rotator cuff) tendon but may also be seen in the quadriceps, Achilles, and patellar tendons.

calcinosis: The deposit of calcium in soft tissue, often seen in the setting of pseudogout.

calcium: An element that is one of the most common minerals for muscle function and bone formation. In ion form, it is crucial for carrying nerve impulses and blood clotting.

calcium pyrophosphate dehydrate (CPPD): A crystal arthropathy in which calcium pyrophosphate dehydrate is deposited into joints, also known as pseudogout. Upon microscopic inspection, the crystals are often rhomboid in shape and weakly positively birefringent.

calipers: An instrument with 2 adjustable arms that is used for measuring the distance between 2 objects, thickness, or diameter.

callus: A thickened area of skin formed due to repetitive friction or pressure, often seen on the hands and feet.

callus formation: Calcium deposits of immature bone formed around fractures during the healing phase.

CAM (controlled ankle movement) boot: A lower extremity brace that encircles the lower leg and looks like a boot. Patients may weight bear through the boot if instructed by their medical providers (*see* Appendix 18).

cam lesion: A form of femoroacetabular impingement in which there is excess bone formation on the superior-lateral portion of the femoral head that contacts the acetabulum when the hip is flexed and internally rotated.

camptodactyly: A congenital anomaly in which one or more fingers is permanently flexed at the proximal interphalangeal joint, often seen in the small finger.

canaliculus: A small duct in the body; in the bone, it refers to the network of hairlike channels that connect the lacunae in bone with one another.

cancellous: A type of bone composed of a porous and spongy structure seen beneath the layer of cortical bone that is less dense in nature.

cancellous screw: A type of screw designed with larger pitch and deeper threads to provide better fixation in cancellous bone.

cannula: A surgical instrument used as a guide that is often inserted with a trocar, which can then be removed to leave the cannula behind.

cannulated: Describes a surgical device with a hollow center that can either be inserted over another piece of equipment or have equipment placed within it. Often used to describe screws that can be inserted over a guide wire or guide pin.

capacitance: Elastic capacity of vessels and organs.

capital epiphysis: The area of growth in the proximal femur that begins at 6 months of age and fuses at maturity. The site of slipped capital femoral epiphysis often seen in obese children.

capitate: The largest carpal bone located in the distal row of carpal bones.

capitellum: A knob-like prominence, often at the end of bones. The most commonly discussed bone is the humeral capitellum, located on the lateral distal humeral condyle that articulates with the radius.

capsule: A fibrous sheath that surrounds a joint.

capsulitis: Inflammation of the lining of the joint.

capsulodesis: Tightening of the joint capsule for the soft tissue to hold the articular surface in alignment and to prevent dislocation.

capsulotomy: Incision of a capsule to obtain access to the joint.

carcinoma: Any of the several kinds of cancerous growths deriving from epithelial cells.

carpal bones: The 8 bones that comprise the wrist (scaphoid, lunate, triquetrum, pisiform, trapezium, trapezoid, capitate, hamate).

carpal tunnel: An anatomic location in the wrist bordered by the transverse carpal ligament, pisiform, hamate, scaphoid, and trapezium, which contains the median nerve and the finger flexor tendons (flexor digitorum superficialis, FDS; flexor digitorum profundus, FDP; flexor pollicis longus, FPL).

carpal tunnel syndrome: Compression of the median nerve within the carpal tunnel that results in pain and tingling over the first 3 fingers (thumb, index, and long fingers) and thenar atrophy.

carpectomy: Surgical removal of the wrist bones, often for deformity or arthritis. Often performed for the proximal row of carpal bones (proximal row carpectomy).

Carter pillow: A foam pillow that holds the arm elevated to reduce swelling, often used in the postoperative period or after reduction of a fracture.

cartilage: Specialized fibrous connective tissue found in various forms throughout the body, including elastic, hyaline, and fibrocartilage.

cast: A rigid dressing used to immobilize a body part to allow for healing. Often composed of fiberglass or plaster and specialized cotton padding (*see* Appendix 17).

cast burn: A skin injury due to heat generated from the hardening of plaster or fiberglass.

cast shoe: A hard-soled shoe placed over the end of the cast so that a patient can bear weight through the cast without eroding the cast.

cast sock: A stockinette used underneath a cast.

cast sore: A skin lesion caused by pressure or abrasion from the cast.

cauda equina: Spinal nerves descending in the spinal column below the level of L2.

cauda equina syndrome: Compression or transection of spinal nerves at the level of the cauda equina that results in loss of bowel and bladder control.

caudal: Away from the head or toward the lower part of a part or structure. *Synonym*: Inferior.

cauterization: Coagulation of blood by the application of chemicals or heat. Electrocautery is often used in surgery to reduce blood loss.

cavus foot: A high arched foot associated with neurologic conditions, including Charcot-Marie-Tooth disease and polio.

cellulitis: An inflammation of connective tissue, especially subcutaneous tissue. Inflammation of tissue around a lesion is characterized by redness, swelling, and tenderness.

cement: A material composed of polymethylmethacrylate (PMMA) that binds 2 surfaces or fills a void. Commonly used in joint replacement procedures or for antibiotic spacers in joint replacement and trauma.

cemented hip replacement: A hip replacement that utilizes implants that are cemented into bone for fixation. This creates 2 different interfaces: bone to cement and cement to prosthesis.

cementless hip replacement: A hip replacement that utilizes implants with porous rough surfaces to allow bony ingrowth or ongrowth to the prosthesis. This creates only one interface: bone and prosthesis.

center edge angle (CEA): On an anterioposterior (AP) view of the pelvis, the angle is formed by drawing a vertical line straight through the femoral head and a line from the center of the femoral head to the lateral edge of the acetabulum. An angle between 25 and 40 degrees is normal, an angle less than 20 degrees may be dysplastic, and an angle greater than 40 degrees may indicate a pincer lesion or overcoverage of the acetabulum. *Synonyms:* Acetabular angle, acetabular index, angle of Wiberg.

centesis: To puncture a cavity to remove fluid.

central cord syndrome: An incomplete spinal cord injury that affects the center portion of the spinal cord, resulting in decreased or absent motor function of the upper extremities. Often due to trauma, ischemia, or hemorrhage.

central nervous system (CNS): Consists of all of the neurons of the brain, brainstem, and spinal cord.

central slip: A fibrous band that extends from the extensor tendon of the finger and inserts into the middle phalanx.

central tendency: The middle or central scores in a distribution.

cephalad: Toward the head or upper portion of a part or structure. *Synonym:* Superior.

cerclage wire: A sterile wire placed around bone to stabilize a fracture. May be used independently or through a plate.

cerebellar ataxia: A broad-based gait with loss of balance due to trauma or disease of the cerebellum.

cerebral palsy (CP): A chronic disease of the central nervous system characterized by impaired muscle coordination and reflexes, associated with premature childbirth and anoxia.

cerebrospinal fluid (CSF): A clear fluid produced in the cranial ventricles that surrounds the spinal cord and brain and provides nutrients.

cervical: Refers to the neck.

cervical collar: A hard or soft collar used to immobilize the cervical spine, either after injury or in the postoperative period (*see* Appendix 18).

cervical vertebrae: Seven neck bones between the skull and thoracic vertebrae that support the head and allow movement.

chamfer: An edge that is beveled, most commonly about 45 degrees. Often refers to the anterior and posterior bone cuts made on the femur in total knee arthroplasties.

chance fracture: A flexion and distraction injury that results in a break in the vertebrae, commonly seen in the thoracolumbar region. The anterior part of the vertebrae is often compressed, and the posterior elements have a transverse fracture through it. Often seen after motor vehicle accidents where flexion of the spine occurs at the level of the lap belt.

Chaput fracture: A pattern where the posterolateral articular surface of the distal tibia is fractured.

Charcot's joint: A joint progressively destroyed due to lack of sensation. Often affects the weight-bearing surfaces of feet, characterized by bone resorption, destruction, and deformity. Patients present with erythema that disappears when the extremity is elevated. Also known as a sequelae of neuropathic arthropathy.

Charcot-Marie-Tooth disease (CMT): An inherited neuropathy that results in the progressive degeneration of peripheral nerves that manifests as muscle loss and loss of sensation. Physical exam findings are commonly foot drop and clawed toes. There are 5 types of CMT, resulting from demyelination or axon malfunction. *Synonyms:* Hereditary motor and sensory neuropathy (HMSN), peroneal muscular atrophy.

charley horse: A colloquial term for a leg cramp or spasm.

Charlson Comorbidity Index (CCI): A measurement that predicts the 10-year mortality for patients with certain comorbidities. Specific diseases are weighted and summed to generate a number, where higher numbers indicate a higher chance of mortality.

Charnley retractor: A self-retaining retraction device used in the hip and spine. Variable arms are connected to the frame to allow retraction at different locations and different depths.

chauffeur's fracture: A break in the radial styloid.

cheilectomy: A surgical excision of an osteophyte at the edge of the first metatarsophalangeal joint in the foot. Commonly used for surgical treatment of early stage hallux rigidus.

chemonucleolysis: A treatment for lumbar disc herniation in which the chemical chymopapain is injected into an intervertebral disc to dissolve it.

chemotherapy: The use of drugs or pharmacologic agents that have a specific and toxic effect on a disease-causing pathogen.

chevron osteotomy: A type of surgical procedure used to treat bunions where a V-shaped bone cut is made into the first metatarsal to realign the bones and correct the hallus valgus.

Chiari procedure: A type of pelvic osteotomy to correct acetabular dysplasia in pediatric patients, in which an osteotomy is performed through the innominate bone of the pelvis and the bone is brought down over the acetabulum to give the femoral head more coverage.

child abuse: Physical, emotional, or sexual ill-treatment of children. Orthopedic manifestations include spiral femur and tibia fractures, metaphyseal corner fractures, posterior rib fractures, and fractures at various stages of healing.

chi-square (χ2): A statistical test used to establish whether frequency differences of categorical variables have occurred on the basis of chance.

chondritis: Inflammation of cartilage.

chondroblast: A chondrocyte progenitor cell that originates from mesenchymal stem cells in the presence of transforming growth factor β (TGF-β).

chondroblastoma: A mostly benign cartilage tumor often seen in the epiphysis or apophysis of long bones. It is most commonly found in the proximal humerus, distal femur, and proximal tibia. *Synonym*: Codman tumor.

chondrocalcinosis: The deposit of calcium within cartilage.

chondroclast: A multinucleated cell that resorbs cartilage.

chondrocyte: A cartilage cell embedded in a lacunae within the matrix of cartilage connective tissue that rarely replicates.

chondrodysplasia: Hereditary condition that results in malformed bone, joint deformities, and dwarfism. Characterized by stippled epiphysis in infancy that disappears by 1 year of age.

chondrofibroma: A benign tumor made of fibrous and cartilaginous tissue. *Synonym*: Chondromyxoma.

chondroitin sulfate: A sulfated glycosaminoglycan (GAG) that comprises connective tissue, especially cartilage. Used as a nutritional supplement thought to protect cartilage.

chondrolysis: The resorption or loss of articular cartilage due to infection or autoimmune diseases.

chondroma: A benign cartilage tumor composed of mature hyaline cartilage. Named based on its location.

chondromalacia: Abnormal softening and fraying of articular cartilage.

chondromyxosarcoma: A malignant tumor composed of cartilage and mucus.

chondroplasty: Surgical repair or débridement of cartilage.

chondrosarcoma: A malignant cartilage tumor. Primary chondrosarcoma arises in the pediatric patient population, and secondary chondrosarcoma is seen in adult patients from preexisting benign conditions, such as osteochondromas or enchondromas.

Chopart amputation: A foot amputation through the midtarsal joint.

chordoma: A rare malignant tumor of the spinal cord arising from remnant notochord most often seen in the cervical and sacral regions of the spine.

chorea: Involuntary dance-like movements of the extremities secondary to central nervous system diseases, such as Huntington disease.

chronic: A slow progression of a condition. *Antonym:* Acute.

circumflex: An arc or circle, often used in naming nerves or vessels that surround a structure (eg, medial and lateral femoral circumflex artery and vein).

claudication: Intermittent pain during exertion caused by insufficient blood supply to the lower extremities from narrowed blood vessels, seen in medical conditions such as atherosclerosis and diabetes.

clavicle: A curved bone that connects the manubrium of the sternum to the acromion of the scapula that has multiple muscle attachments.

claw foot: A pathologic condition in which the foot has an abnormally high arch, often associated with neurologic conditions.

claw hand: A pathologic condition in which the metacarpophalangeal joints are hyperextended and the proximal and distal interphalangeal joints are flexed to look like a claw. Often present in neurological disorders, ulnar nerve lesions, and Volkmann contracture.

claw plate: A surgical device placed on the greater trochanter of the femur and fixed with wires to fix a greater trochanter fracture or osteotomy.

claw toes: A pathologic condition in which the metatarsophalangeal joints are hyperextended and the proximal interphalangeal joints are flexed to look like a claw. Often present in Charcot-Marie-Tooth disease and rheumatoid arthritis.

clear cell chondrosarcoma: A rare, low-grade chondrosarcoma composed of hyaline cartilage and clear cells found in the epiphysis of long bones, especially the proximal femur and humerus.

clonus: Spasmodic alternation of contraction and relaxation of muscle. Often a sign of upper motor neuron lesions, such as strokes or multiple sclerosis.

closed-chain movements: The distal end of a kinematic chain is fixed or stabilized and the proximal end (origin) moves.

closed fracture: A fracture that does not pierce the skin. *Synonym:* Simple fracture.

closed reduction: Placing a fractured bone into an anatomical position with external manipulation without cutting the skin.

closing wedge osteotomy: Removal of a wedge segment of bone to allow the ends of bone to come together in order to realign deformed bone.

clubfoot: A congenital defect of abnormal bone formation in the foot. There are 4 different variations, of which the most common is when the foot is in equinovarus (the soles of the feet face medially and the toes point inferiorly). Clubfoot is often treated conservatively with Ponseti casting and surgically with various releases and reconstructions. *Synonym:* Talipes.

clubhand: Medical condition seen in children in which the hand is displaced. The displacement may be radial or ulnar, with deviation toward the bone that is partially formed or absent. *Synonym:* Talipomanus.

coalition: An abnormal fusion of bones in the foot or hand.

coagulation: The process of blood clot formation.

coagulopathy: A pathological defect in coagulation of the blood.

coaptation splint: A splint used for humeral shaft fractures, where the plaster is wrapped from the base of the neck, around the elbow, and under the axilla and secured with an elastic bandage. Often given a valgus mold to prevent the fracture from displacing (*see* Appendix 17).

Cobb angle: An angle measured from an anterioposterior (AP) spine projection to determine the severity of a spine curvature. A line is drawn from the superior end plate of the apical vertebrae affected by the curve and another line is drawn from the inferior end plate of the inferior vertebrae affected by the curve. The Cobb angle is the angle between the perpendicular lines drawn from the other 2 lines.

Cobb elevator: A surgical instrument composed of a flattened spoon-like end with a narrow, curved edge that is used for stripping ligaments and muscles.

cobra retractor: A surgical instrument that has a flared and bent end that looks like a cobra.

coccydynia: Pain within the coccyx.

coccyx: The distal end of the sacrum composed of 3 to 5 rudimentary fused coccygeal vertebrae. *Synonym*: Tailbone.

cock-up wrist splint: A splint that immobilizes the wrist in an extended position (*see* Appendix 17). May be used in the setting of radial nerve injuries.

codeine: A narcotic medication derived from the opium family used for analgesia.

Codman triangle: A radiographic sign where the periosteum is being lifted by either a tumor (often osteosarcoma) or infection (osteomyelitis).

coefficient of contingency (C): A statistical test used on nominal data to determine correlation.

coefficient of determination (r2): A statistical parameter that determines what proportion of information about y is contained in x.

cogwheel rigidity: A jerky motion that resembles the ratcheted resistance of a gearwheel, commonly seen in Parkinson disease.

Coleman block test: A test to determine hindfoot flexibility in a cavus foot. A block is placed under the lateral portion of the foot with the first metatarsal off of the block. If hindfoot varus corrects, the patient has a flexible deformity; otherwise, the patient has a rigid deformity.

collagen: A fibrous protein in the extracellular matrix and connective tissue that comprises the main supportive structure for skin, tendon, bone, and cartilage. There are many different types of collagen, but over 90% of the collagen within the body is composed of type I, II, and III.

collarbone: A colloquial term for the clavicle.

collateral ligaments: Ligamentous attachments to the side of hinged joints that provide stability and support to joints.

Colles wrist fracture: Fracture of the distal radius with dorsal (or posterior) displacement of the hand. Often caused by a fall onto an outstretched hand.

colonized: Presence of bacteria that causes no local or systemic signs or symptoms.

comminuted fracture: A break in bone resulting in more than 2 fragments.

comorbidity: Having one or more medical diseases. Often used as a measurement of health status.

compartment: A group of muscles separated by fascia layers in the extremities.

compartment syndrome: The compression of nerves, blood vessels, and muscles within a muscle compartment surrounded by fascia. Increased pressure in a compartment greater than 30 mm Hg or pressure that is 30 mm Hg greater than diastolic blood pressure is indicative of compartment syndrome. Most commonly presents with the 5 P's: pain (especially with passive stretch), paresthesia, pallor, paralysis, and pulselessness. This is a true surgical emergency and is surgically treated with fasciotomies.

compensatory curve: The spinal curvature in scoliosis patients that is above and below the major curve.

complete blood count (CBC): A laboratory test that provides the white and red blood cell counts, hemoglobin, hematocrit, and platelets.

compound fracture: A break in bone where one of the ends is visible through skin. Most often referred to as an open fracture.

compression arthrodesis: A joint fusion held by compression, often using plates.

compression dressing: A material used to cover a wound with equal pressure, often used to decrease swelling or tamponade bleeding or wound drainage.

compression fracture: A fracture of the vertebrae only affecting the anterior column where the bone is depressed inferiorly. Often seen in osteoporotic patients after mechanical falls.

compression plate: An orthopedic implant used in internal fixation that increases pressure across 2 ends of bone (fracture or osteotomy) to promote primary healing.

compression therapy: Treatment using devices or techniques that decrease the density of a part of the body through the application of pressure.

computed tomography (CT): A type of radiographical imaging using x-ray technology to construct cross-sectional images of a patient's body, often used to visualize bone (*see* Appendix 22).

concussion: An injury sustained from a blow to the head that results in temporary unconsciousness, confusion, or temporary incapacity. When sustained in an athlete, the player must be removed from the game.

conduction time: The amount of time it takes for an impulse to travel along the course of a nerve.

conduction velocity: A measurement of nerve function measured by the conduction time divided by the distance traveled.

condyle: The rounded end of long bones.

conflict of interest: Situation in which a person may have hidden or other interests (often financial) that conflict with or are inconsistent with providing services to a patient.

congenital: Present or existing at birth.

congenital vertical talus: A cause of rigid flat foot where the navicular bone of the foot is irreducibly dorsally dislocated on the talus. This results in a radiograph where the navicular is dorsally displaced and the talus is vertical. May be due to genetic disease or neurological disorders.

conjoined tendon: A tendon that connects 2 or more muscles to the same location. In the shoulder, the conjoined tendon is composed of the short head of the biceps and the coracobrachialis. In the hip, the conjoined tendon is composed of the superior and inferior gemelli and the obturator internus.

constrained: To limit motion. May refer to orthopedic implants, such as a constrained liner used in a hip and a constrained knee prosthesis that prevents varus and valgus motions.

continuous passive motion (CPM): Device used to passively move a joint through a range of motion. Often used in the postoperative phase after knee surgery to gain early range of motion.

contour: To shape. Often used to shape plates to fit bone or shape rods to fix a skeletal deformity.

contraction: (1) The tightening of a muscle to create stabilization or movement. The development of tension within a muscle or muscle group with or without changes in its overall length. (2) The pulling together of wound edges in the healing process.

contracture: Static shortening of muscle and connective tissue that limits range of motion at a joint.

contraindication: Condition that deems a particular type of treatment undesirable or improper.

contralateral: The opposite side. *Antonym:* Ipsilateral.

contrecoup injury: Usually more extensive damage on the opposite side of the brain from the point of impact during a strike to the head.

control group: In research, a baseline group of patients that is compared to the experimental condition to determine whether there is a difference.

contusion: A bruise.

conus medullaris: The tapered caudal end of the spinal cord before it divides into the cauda equine at the level of L1 to 2.

convulsion: Paroxysms of involuntary muscular contractions and relaxation; a spasm.

coracobrachialis: A muscle that flexes and adducts the shoulder and originates from the coracoid process and inserts in the middle of the humerus.

coracoid: An anterior projection of bone from the scapula that serves as an attachment of multiple ligaments (coracoacromial, coracoclavicular, and coracohumeral ligaments) and muscles (coracobrachialis, pectoralis minor, and biceps).

coronoid process: A triangular portion of bone on the proximal anterior ulna responsible for stabilizing the elbow joint; it resists varus stress and prevents posterior elbow subluxation. Location where the brachialis muscle inserts.

correlation coefficient: A statistical parameter that defines the relationship between 2 or more variables.

cortex: The outermost layer of a structure or organ.

cortical bone: The hard outer layer of bone that provides structure and protection.

cortical defect: A condition in which a portion of cortex is missing, often due to trauma.

cortical screw: A type of screw designed with smaller pitch and shallower threads to provide better fixation in cortical bone. The end of the screw is often blunt, and the fixation is usually through both cortices.

cortisone: A hormone produced in the cortex of the adrenal gland that aids in the regulation of the metabolism of fats, carbohydrates, sodium, potassium, and proteins.

cost–benefit analysis: Process used to evaluate the economic efficiency of new policies and programs by comparing an outcome and the costs required to achieve it.

cost containment: Approach to health care that emphasizes reduced costs.

cost effectiveness: Extent to which funds spent to improve health and well-being reduce overall cost of care.

costochondritis: Inflammation of the cartilage connecting the ribs to the sternum.

coup injury: Brain contusions and lacerations beneath the point of impact when the head is struck.

coxa: The hip or hip joint.

coxa saltans: A condition in which hip flexion and extension causes a snapping sensation. The causes may be extra-articular (iliotibial band/tensor fascia lata/gluteus medius rubbing against the greater trochanter with or without greater trochanteric bursitis) or intra-articular (torn acetabular labrum, ligamentum teres tear, loose bodies, or synovial chondromatosis). *Synonyms:* Snapping hip syndrome, iliopsoas tendinitis, dancer hip.

coxa valgus: A femoral neck-shaft angle of greater than 135 degrees.

coxa vara: A femoral neck-shaft angle of less than 120 degrees.

COX-2 inhibitors: A class of nonsteroidal anti-inflammatory drugs (NSAIDs) that block cyclooxygenase-2 (COX-2) to reduce inflammation. The benefit of this class of drugs is that it is less likely to affect the gastrointestinal system, as opposed to COX inhibitors.

c reactive protein (CRP): An inflammatory marker produced by the liver that is elevated in acute inflammation and infection.

creatinine phosphokinase (CPK): An enzyme in skeletal and cardiac muscle that is elevated when these muscles are damaged. CPK is also elevated in compartment syndrome.

crepitus: Crunching sound or sensation, especially when the 2 ends of bone are rubbing against each other.

crescent sign: A thin, curvilinear radiolucent line seen on x-ray below the articular surface of bone that represents the separation of articular cartilage from subchondral bone due to avascular necrosis.

cross-body test: A physical exam of the shoulder where the arm is adducted across the body in 90 degrees of forward flexion to localize acromioclavicular pathology.

cross-finger flap: A surgical technique of using skin graft from one finger on an adjacent finger.

cross-linked: A chemical reaction where substances are joined to create covalent bonds, in either plastics or proteins. Often used to increase the strength of polyethylene used in orthopedic implants.

crossover sign: A radiographic sign seen on an anteroposterior (AP) projection of the pelvis or the hip that denotes that the patient has acetabular retroversion. This occurs when the line for the anterior wall of the acetabulum crosses or goes medial to the posterior wall acetabular line. This can be associated with a pincer lesion in patients with femoroacetabular impingement (FAI).

cross-sectional research: A research design without experimentation in which a section of the population is examined at a point in time to note possible trends.

cruciate ligaments: Ligaments in the knee (anterior and posterior) that connect the femur to the tibia and prevent anterior and posterior translation.

crutches: A piece of equipment made of metal or wood that looks like a stick with an armrest that supports a patient's weight from the armpit to the floor. Used to assist patients in ambulation and for balance, especially when they have weight bearing restrictions.

cryotherapy: Therapeutic application of cold to provide analgesia and decrease inflammation (eg, ice).

crystal arthropathy: Diseases of the joint that result in crystallization, such as gout and pseudogout.

cubital tunnel: An area on the medial side of the elbow where the ulnar nerve lies and may become compressed. A direct trauma to this area can cause shooting pain down the arm, which is often referred to as striking the funny bone.

cubitus: The elbow joint, or the region between the distal humerus and proximal radius and ulna.

cubitus valgus: A condition when the forearm deviates away from the midline and is often a sequelae after a lateral condyle humerus fracture.

cubitus varus: A condition when the forearm deviates toward the midline and is often a sequelae after a supracondylar humerus fracture. This condition is often cosmetic and rarely reduces function. *Synonym:* Gunstock deformity.

curettage: To scrape and remove tissue and bone to treat tumors, remove infected tissue, and clean the end of fractured bone.

curette: A surgical instrument with a spoon-like end.

curvature: Structural deformity of the spine resulting in scoliosis, kyphoscoliosis, lordosis, or kyphosis.

cutaneous: Relating to the skin.

cutting needle: A type of needle used in suturing, with a sharpened tip to cut through tissue.

cyanosis: Blue discoloration of the skin and mucous membranes due to excessive concentration of reduced hemoglobin in the blood.

cylinder cast: A type of cast applied to the leg that begins proximally at the upper thigh and ends distally at the malleoli. It is placed with the leg in extension and does not incorporate the foot. Patients may bear weight through this cast (*see* Appendix 17).

cyst: A closed sac or pouch with a definite wall that contains fluid, semisolid, or solid material.

cytokine: A soluble factor that provides communication between cells of the immune system, often a growth factor.

cytotoxic: The ability to kill cells.

D

dacron tape: A surgical implant tape made of synthetic polyester (polyethylene terephthalate) used to attach ligaments together or to attach metal to bone.

Dakin solution: An antiseptic solution used to irrigate wounds that consists of sodium hypochloride and boric acid.

Darrach procedure: Removal of the distal ulna to treat distal radioulnar arthritis and distal radioulnar disruption.

death rates: Number of deaths occurring within a specific population during a particular time period, usually in terms of 1000 persons per year.

débridement: Excision of unhealthy or contaminated tissue.

decision analysis: Process used to make health care decisions by utilizing statistical tools, such as multivariate analysis and decision tree analysis.

decompression: Surgical removal of tissue or bone to relieve pressure from an area. For spinal surgery, decompression refers to removing the lamina (laminectomy) to relieve pressure from the spinal cord or nerve roots.

decorticate rigidity: Exaggerated extensor tone of the lower extremities and flexor tone of the upper extremities resulting in abnormal posture due to damage to the brainstem.

decortication: Removing the cortex, or outer layer, of bone. Often used in spinal surgery to provide local autograft for fusion.

decubitus ulcer: Open sore due to lowered circulation in a body part. Usually secondary to prolonged pressure at a bony prominence.

deep tendon reflex (DTR): An involuntary contraction of muscle elicited by percussing a tendon, which travels through a neuron arc through the spinal cord and then stimulates the muscle stretch receptors (*see* Appendix 11). *Synonym*: Myotatic reflex.

Chen AF, ed.
*Quick Reference Dictionary
for Orthopedics (pp 44-53).*
© 2012 Taylor & Francis Group.

deep vein thrombosis (DVT): A blood clot in a deep vein formed at the given site. May be seen in the postoperative state with decreased mobility.

deficiency: The absence or lack of something essential.

degenerative disc disease: The destruction of the intervertebral discs in the spine secondary to age or trauma.

degenerative joint disease (DJD): A type of arthritis that occurs secondary to chronic wear to the cartilage, often due to age or obesity.

degrees of freedom (df): A statistical parameter that determines the number of variables that are free to vary in the final calculation of a statistic.

dehiscence: The abnormal opening of a postsurgical wound along the suture line.

delayed primary closure: Closing a wound after it has been left open for a period of time to allow for initial healing. Often used if a wound is large and may not be closed primarily or after infection to allow appropriate drainage prior to closing the wound.

Delbert classification: A fracture classification system for pediatric hip fractures (*see* Appendix 15).

delirium: Characterized by a confused mental state with changes in attention, hallucinations, delusions, and incoherence. Often seen in elderly individuals in an unfamiliar hospital setting.

delirium tremens (DT): A form of delirium that is often a consequence of excessive alcohol consumption; this acute alcohol withdrawal often appears 72 hours postoperatively and may present with autonomic hyperactivity, tremors, and visual hallucinations.

deltoid ligament: A broad and flat triangular ligament on the medial aspect of the foot that connects the distal tibia to the talus, calcaneus, and navicular.

deltoid muscle: The triangular muscle resting over the superior shoulder that assists with abducting the arm. Its origin is on the acromium, clavicle, and scapular spine, and its insertion is on the deltoid tuberosity of the humerus.

deltoid-pectoral approach: A surgical approach used to expose the glenohumeral joint utilizing the internervous plane between the deltoid (axillary nerve) and pectoralis major (medial and lateral pectoral nerves). The cephalic vein is often used as a marker when trying to find this interval.

deltoid splitting approach: A surgical approach where the deltoid muscle is split to gain access to the proximal humerus. Often used for mini open rotator cuff repairs.

demarcation: Line of separation between viable and nonviable tissue.

dementia: State of deterioration of personality and intellectual abilities, including memory, problem-solving skills, language use, and thinking, that interferes with daily functioning. May be due to brain deterioration.

demineralization: The loss of mineral salts in bone that results in decreased strength of bone.

demyelination: The destruction of myelin. The loss of myelin decreases the conduction velocity of the neural impulse and destroys the white matter of structures within the nervous system. Multiple sclerosis is an example of a demylinating disease.

dendrite: Short processes found on the end of a nerve cell that send or receive information from another neurotransmitter.

Denis classification of vertebral fractures: A fracture classification system of vertebral fractures that divides the vertebrae into 3 columns: (1) anterior: includes the anterior half of the vertebral body and the anterior longitudinal ligament; (2) middle: includes the posterior half of the vertebral body and the posterior longitudinal ligament; and (3) posterior: includes the posterior elements of the vertebrae, including the pedicles, lamina, facet joints, and spinous processes (*see* Appendix 15).

dens: A superior bony projection from the odontoid (C2) that is a pivot point around which the atlas (C1) rotates.

dependent: The region of the body that is closer to the ground and is affected by gravity. May refer to the lower extremities when standing and to the buttocks when laying supine.

dependent edema: Swelling of the lower extremities, especially after standing for long periods of time.

de Quervain disease: Chronic inflammation of the first compartment of the hand that affects the abductor pollicis longus (APL) and extensor pollicis brevis (EPB) tendons. Physical exam finding is a positive Finkelstein test. Treated with splinting, resting, corticosteroid injections, or surgical intervention by excising the tendon.

dermal: Related to the skin or derma. *Synonym:* Skin.

dermatome: An area of the skin that receives cutaneous innervation from one spinal segment.

dermatomyositis: Systemic connective tissue disease characterized by inflammatory and degenerative changes in the skin, leading to symmetric weakness and some atrophy.

dermis: The inner layer of skin in which hair follicles and sweat glands originate; involved in grade II to IV decubitus ulcers.

derotation osteotomy: A bone cut that produces 2 ends of long bone that may be rotated into anatomic alignment and fixed with internal or external fixation.

descriptive statistics: Statistical parameters that summarize the data in quantitative terms, including measurements of central tendency.

desmoid: A benign fibroblast tumor often found in the abdomen. In orthopedics, extra-abdominal desmoid tumors may be found in tendons, muscle, joints, and bone.

developmental dysplasia of the hip (DDH): A congenital condition in which there is incomplete formation of the acetabulum. This results in an unstable hip joint, where the femoral head is partially or fully uncovered by the acetabulum.

dextroscoliosis: A spine curvature to the right.

diabetes: A metabolic disorder in which there is underproduction of insulin or the body no longer responds to insulin that results in high blood sugars. This may present as excessive urination and thirst and may progress to sensation loss in the extremities that can lead to neurogenic arthropathy (destruction of a joint).

diagnosis-related groups (DRG): Classifications of illnesses and injuries that are used as the basis for prospective payments to hospitals under Medicare and other insurers.

dial test: A test performed on the knee to assess the stability of the posterolateral corner (PLC) and the posterior cruciate ligament (PCL). The patient is placed supine on the table and the lower leg is externally rotated at 30 and 90 degrees. If there is an isolated PLC injury, the dial test will be positive at 30 degrees, and if there is a combined PLC and PCL injury, the dial test will be positive at 90 degrees. A positive test is when there is greater than 10 degrees of movement compared to the contralateral leg.

diaphysis: The shaft of long bones.

diastasis: Abnormal separation of 2 bones without a fracture.

diastrophic dysplasia: A congenital anomaly characterized by short arms and legs, often associated with cleft palate and clubfeet.

Diclofenac: A type of nonsteroidal anti-inflammatory drug (NSAID) that is a cyclooxygenase (COX) inhibitor. Its chemical name is 2-(2,6-dichloranilino) phenylacetic acid (*see* Appendix 19).

didactylism: A congenital anomaly in which there are only 2 digits on the hand and/or feet.

diffuse: Spread out or dispersed; not concentrated.

diffuse idiopathic skeletal hyperostosis (DISH): Calcification of the tendons attached to the spine that results in ossification of the spine. Presents with nonmarginal syndesmophytes. Also known as Forestier disease.

digit: A finger or a toe.

digital block: A local anesthetic administered to a finger to temporarily decrease sensation.

diplegia: Paralysis involving 2 extremities on both sides of the body.

diplomyelia: A congenital anomaly in which the spinal cord is duplicated (dural sac and nerve roots) that often results in loss of function below the duplication. Often associated with spina bifida.

disarticulation: Amputation of a limb through a joint. Does not require the cutting of bone, which reduces bleeding.

disc: A fibrocartilaginous structure between vertebral bodies that acts as a cushion. The most well known are the intervertebral discs.

discitis: Inflammation within an intervertebral disc in the spine due to infection. X-rays may show intervertebral disc narrowing and destruction, with indistinct adjacent endplates. Magnetic resonance imaging (MRI) shows decreased marrow intensity on T1-weighted images and increased marrow intensity on T2-weighted images due to edema.

disclosure: The act of revealing information. Often refers to a financial disclosure by an individual who receives monetary funding from a specified source.

discoid lateral meniscus: A congenital anomaly of the lateral meniscus in which the meniscus is thickened and presents with a fuller cresent shape. These anatomic variant menisci are more prone to tears, due to the anatomical shape, decreased blood supply, and possibly weaker capsular attachment. An asymptomatic discoid meniscus does not require treatment and the prognosis is generally good.

disease: Deviation from the norm of measureable biological variables as defined by the biomedical system; refers to abnormalities of structure and function in body organs and systems.

disectomy: Surgical removal of a portion of or the entire intervertebral disc.

dislocation: Displacement of a bone from a joint with tearing of ligaments, tendons, and/or articular cartilage. Requires closed or open reduction to restore the anatomical position.

displaced fracture: A fracture pattern in which the bones are no longer in anatomic alignment.

dissect: To surgically separate tissue using instruments or hands.

distal: An anatomical position further away from the trunk.

distal femoral replacement (DFR): A replacement of the distal femur with a megaprosthesis due to tumor, total knee arthroplasty revisions, or fracture.

distal radioulnar joint (DRUJ): The distal articulation of the radius and ulna near the wrist. Must assess stability of the DRUJ after a distal radius fracture.

distend: To fill an area with fluid or gas. After arthroscopic surgery, the joint (knee, hip, shoulder, etc) is often distended with water.

distraction: Linear separation of joint surfaces without ligamentous rupture until the 2 ends are no longer in contact with one another.

distribution: A statistical term used to describe a population showing the observed or theoretical frequency of occurrence.

dog ear: A redundant corner of skin, often due to an uneven closure, or redundancy of other tissue.

donor site: The location from which graft is removed. Most commonly from oneself (eg, skin graft taken from the upper thigh).

Doppler ultrasound: A noninvasive imaging technique that uses ultrasonic sound waves to measure blood flow. Used to diagnose blockages in the artery or vein (deep vein thrombosis).

dormant: Time period when a disease remains inactive.

dorsal: An anatomic position located toward the back. *Synonym*: Posterior. *Antonym*: Volar.

dorsal column tracts: Afferent ipsilateral ascending tracts for fine discriminative touch, vibratory sense, and kinesthesia.

dorsal splint: A splint where plaster is applied to the dorsal aspect of the hand and secured with an elastic bandage to prevent full extension of the wrist or any of the finger joints (*see* Appendix 17).

dorsiflexion: Bending the hand backwards (opposite of palmar or volar flexion) or the foot upwards (opposite of plantarflexion).

double-blind study: An experiment conducted in which both the individuals and the researchers do not know whether an intervention was administered, which reduces experimental error.

double innominate osteotomy: A pelvic osteotomy used to correct developmental dysplasia of the hip where a bone cut is made between the ilium and ischium or ilium and pubis to change the location of the acetabulum to better cover the femoral head.

double joint: When a person has very flexible joints, often occurring in the legs, arms, and fingers. Does not refer to a condition in which an individual actually has 2 joints in one location.

Down syndrome: A genetic condition in which there are 3 copies of chromosome 21. Patients present with atlantoaxial instability, hyperelasticity, mental retardation, and cardiac disease. *Synonym:* Trisomy 21.

drain: A surgical implant that removes fluid from a wound or cavity.

drainage: Fluid that comes from a wound or surgical site.

drawer sign: A physical exam test in which the hip is flexed to 45 degrees, the knee is flexed to 90 degrees, and an anterior or posterior stress is placed on the tibia. If the tibia subluxes anteriorly, it is a positive anterior drawer sign indicating damage to the anterior cruciate ligament; if the tibia subluxes posteriorly, it is a positive posterior drawer sign indicating damage to the posterior cruciate ligament.

drill: An instrument used to bore holes in bone prior to placing screws.

drill guide: A hollow surgical instrument used to direct a drill in a specific direction. May be held by hand or locked into a plate, depending on the screw being used.

dual-emission x-ray absorptiometry (DEXA) scan: A method of measuring bone mineral density by x-ray to determine whether a patient is osteopenic (T-score between −1 and −2.5) or osteoporotic (T-score less than −2.5).

Duchenne-Erb paralysis: Neuropraxia of the muscles of the shoulder commonly affecting the supraspinatus and infraspinatus muscles, which are innervated by the suprascaular nerve that is fixed at Erb's point (suprascapular notch). May also affect the axillary and musculocutaneous nerve. This is secondary to traction on the brachial plexus when being delivered through the pelvic canal.

Duchenne muscular dystrophy (DMD): A hereditary X-linked condition due to a mutation of the dystrophin gene that results in progressive muscle weakness that starts in the proximal lower extremities and spreads to the rest of the body.

duck waddle test: A test used to determine the presence of a meniscal tear, where knee pain is elicited when a patient is asked to squat and then ambulate with the knees internally and externally rotated.

Dunn view: A technique to capture radiographs of the hip to evaluate for femoroacetabular impingement. The patient is supine and the hip is placed in neutral rotation, 90 degrees hip flexion, and 20 degrees abduction. May be modified to 45 degrees hip flexion.

Dupuytren contracture: A fixed flexion contracture of the palmar aponeurosis that forms nodules and cords due to the increased production of fibroblasts. Also known as Viking disease. May be treated either with the drug collagenase or by surgical excision of the fibrous tissue.

dura: The outermost covering over the spinal cord and brain. May be torn during spinal surgery, as indicated by a cerebrospinal fluid (CSF) leak.

durable medical equipment (DME): Medical equipment for patients to use at home to aid with activities of daily living.

Dwyer calcaneal osteomy: A closing wedge osteomy performed in the calcaneus to correct varus in a cavovarus foot.

dynamic compression plate (DCP): A plate with offset screw holes that allows compression at the fracture site when the screws are tightened.

dynamic splint: Orthosis that allows controlled movements at various joints; tension is applied to encourage particular movements.

dynamic tendon transfer: Moving one tendon to another location to supplement an existing or deficient tendon.

dynamometer: An instrument that measures muscular power. Used most commonly to assess grip strength.

dysesthesia: Sensation of "pins and needles" such as that experienced when one's extremity "goes to sleep." Manifested by unpleasant or painful touch perceptions, hyperalgesia. Commonly seen in multiple sclerosis patients.

dyskinesia: Abnormal voluntary movements, often secondary to neurologic conditions such as cerebral palsy (CP) and Parkinson's disease.

dysmorphia: An abnormal shape.

dysmyotonia: An abnormal muscle tone; may be increased (hypertonic) or decreased (hypotonic).

dysostosis: The malformation of bones, often seen in mucopolysaccharidosis.

dysplasia: An abnormality of growth in soft tissue or organs due to a proliferation of cells.

dystonia: Abnormal tension across muscles or soft tissues. In the neck, it is described by cervical dystonia or torticollis, where there is abnormal tension of the sternocleidomastoid muscle.

dystrophy: Disorders characterized by wasting away of an organ or tissue in the body.

E

eburnation: A pathological change where the subchondral bone in a joint is converted to a dense and smooth surface that resembles ivory due to increased wear from osteoarthritis.

eccentric contraction: Muscular contraction during which the muscle generates tension while lengthening. Eccentric exercise occurs mainly in stabilizing the body against gravity.

ecchymosis: Purple discoloration of the skin due to bleeding below the skin surface, often due to trauma. Also known as bruising.

ectoderm: Layer of cells that develop from the inner cell mass of the blastocyst. This layer eventually develops into the outer surface of the skin, nails, part of teeth, lens of the eye, the inner ear, and the central nervous system.

edema: Accumulation of large amounts of fluid in the tissues of the body.

Edwards' syndrome: A cogenital syndrome where patients have trisomy 18 that is characterized by multiple physical malformations and mental retardation. Patients are often born with small heads and jaws, low birth weight, heart and kidney malformations, clenched fists, and malformed feet.

efferent: Conducting away from a structure, such as a nerve or a blood vessel.

effusion: Escape of fluid into a joint or cavity.

Ehlers-Danlos syndrome: A hereditary connective tissue disorder caused by a defect in collagen (type I and III) synthesis that results in hyperelastic joints, skin, and ligaments.

elastic cartilage: The cartilage with the most elastic fibers, making it the most flexible cartilage. Found in the larynx, epiglottis, and outer ear.

elasticity: The amount of tissue force produced when a tissue is deformed and held at a given length.

electrocautery: A surgical device that uses electric current to burn blood vessels to stop bleeding.

electromagnetism: The use of an electromagnetic field to stimulate bone healing. Offered as an external device called a bone stimulator.

electromyography (EMG): The examining and recording of the electrical activity of a muscle (*see* Appendix 23).

embolism: Sudden blocking of an artery or vein by a clot of material from another source brought to the site through the bloodstream (eg, pulmonary embolism traveling from a deep vein thrombosis).

emetic: Drug that promotes vomiting.

enchondroma: A chondroma located within bone.

enchondromatosis: Multiple benign cartilage tumors. Also known as Ollier disease. When associated with multiple hamartomas (benign blood vessels), it is called Maffucci syndrome.

Ender nail: A flexible metal rod placed in the medullary canal used to fix long bones.

endogenous: Growing from within. Developing or originating within the organism.

endoprosthesis: An orthotic artificial device placed inside the body used to replace a missing body part.

endosteum: A thin vascular layer of tissue that lines the medullary canal of long bone.

end point: A sensation in the hands of a clinician at the extremes of range of motion. Also used to determine whether ligamentous laxity is present.

enthesis: The location of tendon attachment to bone.

enthesitis: Inflammation of the tendon–bone junction, often seen in ankylosing spondylitis.

enthesopathy: An erosion of the tendon attachment to bone due to inflammation.

entrapment: To compress a nerve or vessel with surrounding soft tissue or bone.

enucleate: To remove an item in one piece.

eosinophilic granuloma: An older term to denote a unifocal form of Langerhans cell histiocytosis that is often seen on radiograph with a solitary lytic lesion in the skull or spine. Normally does not have any extraskeletal involvement. *Synonym*: Hand-Schüller-Christian disease, Letterer-Siwe disease.

epicondylar: Prominent bone on the medial and lateral sides of some long bones, such as the distal humerus and distal femur.

epicondylar axis: The line by which one may judge rotation of the femur and the placement of the femoral component for a total knee arthroplasty.

epicondylitis: Inflammation of the soft tissue attached to the epicondyles. Lateral epicondylitis of the humerus is also known as tennis elbow, and medial epicondylitis of the humerus is known as golfer's elbow.

epidemiology: A study of the relationships between the various factors determining the frequency and distribution of diseases in a human environment. Science concerned with factors, causes, and remediation as related to the distribution of disease, injury, and other health-related events.

epidermis: The outer layer of skin.

epidural: Anesthesia injected into the space of the spine outside of the dura mater where the spine nerve roots lie. This can produce loss of sensation from the abdomen to the toes and lasts for approximately 2 hours.

epinephrine: A hormone secreted by the adrenal medulla in response to splanchnic stimulation and stored in the chromaffin granules, being released predominantly in response to hypoglycemia. It increases blood pressure, stimulates heart muscle, accelerates the heart rate, and increases cardiac output. Used in the hospital setting to increase blood pressure.

epiphysiodesis: Surgical destruction of the growth plate in bones to prevent further growth, either by curettage or surgical fixation with implants.

epiphyseal plate: An area of cartilage between the epiphysis and metaphysis where the bone grows. *Synonym*: Growth plate, physis.

epiphyseal scar: A radiopaque band seen at the juncture of the epiphysis and metaphysis indicative of a closed physis when a patient is skeletally mature.

epiphysis: The end of long bones.

epithelialization: Regeneration of the epidermis across a wound surface.

eponychium: The skin that covers a portion of the base of the nail, commonly known as the cuticle.

Epstein classification: A classification system for anterior hip dislocations (*see* Appendix 15).

equinovarus: Deformity of the foot in which the foot is pointing inwards (varus) and downwards (equinus); clubfoot.

equinus: Plantarflexion of the foot, either due to positioning or anatomic anomaly in which the gastrocnemius and soleus are shortened. Results in toe walking.

erosion: An area of tissue erosion secondary to ulceration, inflammation, or trauma.

erythema: Redness of the skin due to infection, burn, or injury.

erythrocyte: Red blood cell that contains hemoglobin, an oxygen-carrying pigment responsible for the red color of blood.

erythrocyte sedimentation rate (ESR): A measurement of inflammation determined by the rate at which erythrocytes settle to the bottom of a tube in one hour. An ESR greater than 100 mm/hour is often indicative of an infection or an active inflammatory condition. Also known as sed rate.

eschar: Thick, leathery, necrotic tissue; devitalized tissue; a slough produced by burning or by a corrosive application.

Escherichia coli (*E coli*)*:* A gram-negative bacteria that is native to the gastrointestinal flora. It is commonly found in urinary tract infections and diarrhea.

Esmarch bandage: An elastic band used to exsanguinate a limb prior to inflating a tourniquet.

Essex-Lopresti fractures: (1) Fracture of the radial head with concomitant dislocation of the distal radioulnar joint and interosseous membrane disruption. (2) Fracture of the calcaneus described as joint depression or tongue type.

etiology: Dealing with the causes of disease.

etodolac: A type of nonsteroidal anti-inflammatory drug (NSAID) that is able to inhibit cyclooxygenase (COX) but is more selective for inhibiting COX-2.

eversion: Turning outwards.

evidence-based medicine (EBM): The practice of medicine founded on research that supports its effectiveness.

Ewing sarcoma: A malignant bone tumor often found in the pelvis, femur, humerus, and clavicle. It mostly affects teenage males and is defined by a genetic translocation between chromosomes 11 and 22 (t[11;22]). Ewing's sarcoma is histologically characterized by multiple round blue cells that stain positive for CD99.

exacerbation: Increase in the severity of a disease or any of its symptoms.

exam under anesthesia (EUA): A physical exam on an anesthetized patient to assess for joint laxity and true range of motion.

excise: To surgically remove tissue, including bone, muscle, tumor, or other tissues.

excoriation: An area of deep abrasion that tears off a portion of skin, often due to severe scratching.

excretion: Process through which metabolites of drugs (and active drug itself) are eliminated from the body through urine and feces, evaporation from skin, exhalation from lungs, and secretion into saliva.

Exertional Compartment Syndrome: A medical condition in which exercise and repetitive activities increase pressures within the extremities. Patients may present with pain and/or weakness. Often a chronic condition that is commonly found in the lower extremities. May require surgical intervention (ie, fasciotomies).

exogenous: Growing by additions to the outside. Developed or originating outside the organism.

exostosis: Benign tumor growth with cartilage caps found at the long end of bone.

extended trochanteric osteotomy (ETO): A cut in the bone that extends from the greater trochanter down the femur often used to remove a well-fixed femoral implant.

extension: Straightening of a body part.

extensor: A muscle that straightens a joint from flexion.

extensor carpi ulnaris (ECU): A muscle that extends and ulnarly deviates the wrist. It originates from the lateral epicondyle of the humerus and insets on the base of the fifth metacarpal.

extensor compartments of the wrist: The 6 compartments of the wrist that contribute to extension numbered from the radial to the ulnar side. The compartments are as follows: (1) extensor pollicis brevis (EPB) and abductor pollicis longus (APL), (2) extensor carpi radialis longus (ECRL) and extensor carpi radialis brevis (ECRB), (3) extensor pollicis longus (EPL), (4) extensor indicis propius (EIP) and extensor digitorum muscle, (5) extensor digiti minimi (EDM), and (6) extensor carpi ulnaris (ECU).

extensor digiti minimi (EDM): A muscle that extends the small finger. It originates at the lateral epicondyle of the humerus and inserts at the distal phalanx of the small finger.

extensor digitorum: A muscle that extends the digit. It originates in the lateral epicondyle and inserts in the sagittal bands and central slip of the distal phalanxes of the index, long, ring, and small fingers.

extensor digitorum brevis (EDB): A muscle that extends the great toe. It originates from the dorsal calcaneus and inserts in the base of the proximal phalanx of the great toe.

extensor digitorum longus (EDL): A muscle in the anterior compartment of the leg with 4 tendon insertions that dorsiflexes and extends the lateral 4 toes. It originates from the lateral tibia condyle and proximal fibula and inserts at the base of the middle and distal phalanges of the 4 toes (besides the great toe).

extensor hallucis brevis (EHB): A muscle that extends the 4 lateral toes. It originates from the dorsal calcaneus and inserts at the base of the proximal phalanx of the 4 lateral toes.

extensor hallucis longus (EHL): A muscle in the anterior compartment of the leg that dorxiflexes and extends the great toe. It originates from the medial fibula and interosseous membrane and inserts in the base of the distal phalanx of the great toe.

extensor lag: An inability to fully extend the knee to 0 degrees due to weakening or lengthening of the quadriceps muscle.

extensor pollicis brevis (EPB): A muscle that extends the thumb at the metacarpophalangeal joint. It originates at the posterior radius and inserts at the base of the proximal phalanx of the thumb.

extensor pollicis longus (EPL): A muscle that extends the thumb at the interphalangeal joint. It originates at the posterior ulna and inserts at the base of the thumb of the distal phalanx.

external fixation: Use of pins placed from outside the skin and held together in a rigid frame with bars to hold a fracture in alignment.

external validity: The degree to which an experimental finding is predictable to the population at large.

extra-articular fracture: A fracture that does not involve the articular surface.

extramedullary: Outside of the medullary or marrow canal. May refer to guides used in arthroplasty surgery that do not enter the medullary canal.

extremity: An arm (upper extremity) or leg (lower extremity).

extrinsic: Coming from or originating from outside.

extrusion: Bulging of muscle, bone, or other tissue outside of the anatomically normal space.

exudate: Material, such as fluid, cells, or cellular debris, that has escaped from blood vessels and been deposited in tissues or on tissue surfaces, usually as a result of inflammation. An exudate, in contrast to a transudate, is characterized by a high content of protein, cells, or solid materials derived from cells and is often accumulated in wounds. May contain serum, cellular debris, bacteria, and/or leukocytes.

fabella: Small sesamoid bone within the tendon of the lateral head of the gastrocnemius muscle that may be confused with a loose body or osteophyte.

FABER (flexion, abduction, external rotation) sign: A physical exam in which the hip and knee are flexed and the hip is abducted and externally rotated. Pain with this maneuver indicates that there is pathology of the hip joint or sacroiliac joint. Also known as the Patrick test and the figure-4 test.

facet: The articulation between vertebrae that allows motion in the spine. Each vertebra is composed of 2 superior and 2 inferior facets.

facilitation: To reinforce an activity by repetitively stimulating it. Used after muscle or tendon transfers to "teach" a new task to the muscle.

factor analysis: Statistical test that examines the relationships of many variables and their contribution to the total set of variables.

false negative: Statistical research term indicating the rate of negative results on a diagnostic test when disease was actually present.

false positive: Statistical research term indicating the rate of positive results on a diagnostic test when no disease was actually present.

fan sign: A physical exam sign of neurological deficit where stroking of the plantar surface of the foot results in the toes spreading apart to look like a fan.

fascia: A layer of connective tissue covering, supporting, or connecting the muscles or inner organs of the body.

fascicle: A bunch of fibers (nerves or muscles) surrounded by a layer of thin connective tissue.

fasciculation: A small local contract of muscles, visible through the skin, representing a spontaneous discharge of a number of fibers innervated by a single motor nerve filament.

fasciitis: Inflammation of fascia.

fasciotomy: A surgical procedure in which the fascia is incised to relieve pressure within a compartment.

fat emboli: Embolus formed by an ester of glycerol within fatty acids, which causes a clot in the circulatory system and results in vessel obstruction. Often seen after reaming of intramedullary canals, where the fat in bone marrow is displaced.

fatigue fracture: A hairline break in the bone due to repetitive stress that may not be seen on plain x-ray and may have to be diagnosed by magnetic resonance imaging (MRI).

fat pad sign: A radiolucent area seen on x-ray where fat is noted around bone. It is physiologic when seen in the anterior elbow but is pathologic for a fracture when seen at the posterior distal humerus. Fat from the bone marrow may escape from the fracture site and elevate the soft tissue to produce this sign.

felon: A soft tissue infection at the end of a finger that produces purulent material. *Synonym*: Whitlow.

femoral nerve block: A regional delivery of local anesthetic agent that reduces pain and sensation in the anterior and medial thigh (femoral nerve distribution).

femoroacetabular impingement (FAI): A condition in which the femur and the acetabulum have abnormal contact due to overgrowth of the femur (cam lesion) or acetabulum (pincer lesion) that produces damage to the articular cartilage or labrum.

fenestra: An opening made in bone or fascia.

fiberglass: A material made of glass fibers within a resin matrix that is activated by water and used for casting because it can be molded and is lightweight.

fibril: A small muscle fiber or nerve.

fibrillation: Small, local involuntary muscle contraction.

fibrin: An insoluble protein formed from fibrinogen by the action of thrombin, as in the clotting of blood. Fibrin forms the essential portion of a blood clot.

fibroblast: Chief cell of connective tissue responsible for producing collagen to form the fibrous tissues of the body, such as tendons and ligaments.

fibroblast growth factor (FGF): A family of protein growth factors that contribute to wound healing, angiogenesis, and embryonic development.

fibroblast growth factor receptor (FGFR): Receptors to the FGF family. When mutated it may result in multiple connective tissue disorders, including achondroplasia and Apert syndrome.

fibrocartilage: A tough cartilage made of numerous and thick bundles of collagen that is physiologic in meniscus but pathologic when it replaces defects in hyaline cartilage.

fibrocortical defect: A benign fibrous bone lesion found in the metaphysis of long bones in children.

fibrocyte: A fibroblast that is not actively producing collagen.

fibroma: A benign tumor composed of fibrous connective tissue.

fibromatosis: Multiple benign fibromas found in the hands or plantar surfaces of feet that may lead to contracture and pain.

fibromyalgia: A chronic pain condition characterized by tenderness at specific trigger points.

fibrosarcoma: A malignant tumor that arises from the fibrous tissue of bone, composed of fibroblasts or undifferentiated anaplastic spindle cells.

fibrosis: Formation of fibrous tissue.

fibula: The smaller of the 2 bones on the lateral part of the lower leg that articulates with the tibia and talus.

fibular hemimelia: Congenital absence of all or part of the fibula, associated with a shortened femur and the absence of the third, fourth, and/or fifth metatarsals.

Fielding classification: A fracture classification system for subtrochanteric femur fractures based on the distance from the lesser trochanter of the femur (*see* Appendix 15).

figure 8 harness: A brace used to treat clavicle fractures that keep the shoulders extended (*see* Appendix 18).

filtered exhaust helmets: Helmets often worn by surgeons who perform hip and knee arthroplasty surgery that look like space suits and are used to limit the amount of airborne contaminants produced by humans.

filum terminale syndrome: A condition in which the conus medullaris becomes tethered so that the cord is placed under tension, which can cause paralysis of the lower extremities and loss of bowel and bladder habits. May occur with the closure of spina bifida.

finger trap: An orthopedic device placed on the fingers to pull traction on the hand. Often used to aid distal radius fracture reduction, or used to distract the wrist when perfoming wrist arthroscopies.

Finkelstein test: A physical example test for de Quervain disease or tendonitis of the abductor pollicus longus (APL) in which the examiner holds the patient's hand as if going to shake it, then deviates ulnarly to see whether pain is elicited over the radial side of the wrist.

fishmouth amputation: A surgical technique in which the soft tissue at the distal end of an amputation is made to look like a fish mouth to provide ample soft tissue for closure.

fissure: Any cleft or groove.

fistula: Abnormal passage or tube-like duct connecting 2 organs together or from a normal cavity to the body surface.

fixation: A surgical technique to immobilize bones to one another using plates and screws or other orthopedic devices.

flaccid: Muscle without tone, often seen in cerebral palsy.

flaccidity: State of low tone in the muscle that produces weak and floppy limbs.

flail: Used to describe a limb without muscle control. May be used to describe a badly fractured limb that has no structural integrity or a fractured rib cage that moves independently from the chest wall.

flap: In surgery, refers to an area of tissue that can be elevated or moved to cover an area deficient of soft tissue.

flatfoot deformity: An acquired or congenital condition in which there is a loss of the medial longitudinal arch. Infants and toddlers often have minimal arches, which subsequently develop over time. In adults, the flat foot may be fixed or flexible. Flexible deformities are often due to posterior tibial tendon dysfunction and the heel will correct out of valgus when the patient stands on his or her toes; rigid deformities will not correct. Also known as pes planus.

flexion: Act of bending a body part.

flexion contracture: When a joint is fixed in flexion and cannot be corrected by physical manipulation.

flexor carpi radialis (FCR): A muscle that flexes and radially deviates the wrist. It originates from the medial epicondyle and inserts in the base of the second and third metacarpals.

flexor carpi ulnaris (FCU): A muscle that flexes and ulnarly deviates the wrist. It originates from the medial epicondyle of the posterior ulna and inserts in the pisiform, hook of the hamate, and the fifth metacarpal.

flexor digiti minimi brevis (FDMB): A muscle that flexes the small toe. It originates at the base of the fifth metatarsal and inserts in the base of the proximal phalanx of the small toe.

flexor digitorum brevis (FDB): A muscle that flexes the lateral 4 toes. It originates from the calcaneal tuberosity and inserts in the middle phalanges of the lateral 4 toes.

flexor digitorum longus (FDL): A muscle in the deep compartment of the leg that plantarflexes the second through fifth toes. It originates from the posterior tibia and inserts in the bases of the distal phalanges of the lateral 4 toes.

flexor digitorum profundus (FDP): A muscle that flexes the distal interphalangeal (DIP) joint. It originates from the anterior ulna and interosseous membrane and inserts in the distal phalanx of the index, long, ring, and small fingers.

flexor digitorum superficialis (FDS): A muscle that flexes the proximal interphalangeal (PIP) joint. It originates from the medial epicondyle, coronoid process, and anteroproximal radius. It inserts in the middle phalanges of the index, long, ring, and small fingers.

flexor hallucis brevis (FHB): A muscle that assists with flexing the great toe. It originates from the cuboid and the lateral cuneiform and inserts in the proximal phalanx of the great toe.

flexor hallucis longus (FHL): A muscle in the deep compartment of the leg that plantarflexes the great toe. It originates from the posterior fibula and inserts at the base of the distal phalanx of the great toe.

flexor pollicis brevis (FPB): A muscle that causes the thumb to flex at the metacarpophalangeal joint. It originates from the trapezium and inserts at the base of the proximal phalanx of the thumb.

flexor pollicis longus (FPL): A muscle that flexes the thumb at the interphalangeal joint. It originates from the anterior radius and coronoid process and inserts in the distal phalanx of the thumb.

flexor retinaculum: A fascial sheath across the volar surface of the wrist that contains the flexor tendons and acts as a pulley.

floating ribs: The inferior 2 ribs (11th and 12th ribs) that are not attached to the sternum, which gives them the appearance of floating.

floppy baby syndrome: Decreased muscle tone and movement in a newborn that may be due to muscular dystrophy or cerebral palsy.

fluctuance: A compressible, boggy, and mobile area of tissue indicative of a fluid collection below the skin.

fluoroscopy: X-ray often taken intraoperatively and displayed on a live monitor. May be single picture or continuous.

foot drop: The inability to dorsiflex the foot due to paralysis or absence of muscles within the anterior compartment of the leg.

foramen: A natural opening or hole in bone.

foraminal stenosis: Narrowing of the bony openings from which nerve roots exit the spine, which results in compression and irritation to the nerve roots.

force: Product of mass and acceleration; a kinematic measurement that encompasses the amount of matter, velocity, and its rate of change of velocity; also, strength, energy, and power.

forceps: A type of handheld surgical instrument that is used to grasp and hold objects. A colloquial term used for forceps is tweezers, but this term is not often used in the operating room.

forefoot: The portion of the foot distal to the cuneiform bones.

foreign body (FB): Any object found within the body that is not naturally produced by the body.

forequarter amputation: A surgical procedure in which the arm is removed from the shoulder.

fossa: A cavity or depression in bone.

fovea: The area of the femoral head where the ligamentum teres attaches the femoral head to the acetabulum.

fracture (fx): A broken bone.

fracture-dislocation: Broken bones in conjunction with a dislocated joint.

frame: An object that gives an item structure, such as for holding patients in certain positions.

free radicals: Any molecule that contains one or more unpaired electrons. Accelerates the oxidative process.

friable: Tissue that falls apart easily.

friction band syndrome: Lateral knee pain produced by irritation to and inflammation of the iliotibial band (ITB) as it crosses the knee joint.

Friedreich ataxia: A hereditary condition that causes progressive degeneration of the upper motor neurons that results in gait disturbances (ataxia), contractures, and paralysis.

Frölich syndrome: A disease characterized by obesity and delayed development of secondary sexual characteristics that may be seen in patients with capital femoral epiphysis. Also known as adiposogenital dystrophy and Launois-Cleret syndrome.

Froment sign: A weak pinch between the index finger and distal phalanx of the thumb, which is indicative of ulnar nerve palsy. When the adductor pollicis is unable to perform a pinch due to ulnar nerve palsy, the interphalangeal (IP) joint of the thumb hyperflexes to pinch.

frozen shoulder: Adhesive capsulitis of the shoulder.

fulcrum: The entity on which a lever moves; the intermediate point of force application of a 3- or 4-point bending construction.

full-thickness skin graft (FTSG): A skin graft that includes the epidermis and dermis without removing subcutaneous tissue.

full weight bearing (FWB): Allowed to bear the entire weight of the body on the extremity specified.

functional mobility: Moving from one position or place to another, such as in-bed mobility, wheelchair mobility, and transfers; performing functional ambulation; and transporting objects. The ability to perform functional activities and tasks without restriction.

funny bone: Colloquial term for the region of the medial epicondyle on the distal humerus where the ulnar nerve may experience direct trauma, which results in a tingling sensation down to the ring and small fingers in the hand.

fusion: A surgical procedure by which 2 articulating surfaces of a joint are united. *Synonym*: Arthrodesis.

G

gadolinium (Gd): A commonly used magnetic resonance imaging (MRI) contrast agent, either intravenous, intra-arterial, or intra-articular. Patients with renal disease may need to be pretreated prior to administering gadolinium contrast.

gait: The manner in which a person walks, characterized by rhythm, cadence, step, stride, and speed. The gait cycle is defined by the stance phase and swing phase.

Galeazzi fracture: A fracture pattern in the forearm where the distal third of the radius is fractured with an associated dislocation of the distal radioulnar joint (DRUJ).

Galeazzi sign: A test in infants to determine leg length discrepancy or hip dislocation. The patient is placed supine on the table with the knees flexed and plantar surface of the feet on the table. The knee that is lower either has a hip dislocation or is shorter than the contralateral limb. *Synonym*: Allis test.

gamekeeper thumb: A condition in which the ulnar collateral ligament on the metacarpophalangeal joint of the thumb is ruptured.

ganglion: A mass of nerve cells serving as a center from which impulses are transmitted.

ganglion cyst: A sac of fluid arising from the joint capsule or a tendon sheath.

gangliosidosis: An autosomal recessive condition in which there is an abnormal accumulation of lipids, specifically gangliosides, in the brain and nerve tissues that causes progressive motor and mental deterioration and often death in early childhood. Found in higher prevalence in patients of eastern European Jewish descent.

gangrene: Decay of tissue in a part of the body where the blood supply is obstructed by disease or injury.

garden classification: A fracture classification system for femoral neck fractures based on the amount of valgus impaction (*see* Appendix 15).

Gardner-Wells tongs: A device used to fix the head in a set position for spinal traction or for performing surgery. Sharp pins are placed in both sides of the skull with a U-shaped metal arch connecting them from which traction can be applied.

Garth view: A technique to capture radiographs of the glenohumeral (GH) joint. The patient is seated with the arm adducted and internally rotated, where the hand is placed over the heart. The beam is directed 45 degrees caudal and 45 degrees cephalad.

Gartland classification: A fracture classification system for extension type supracondylar humerus fractures based on the amount of displacement (*see* Appendix 15).

gastrocsoleus: The muscles in the posterior compartment of the leg composed of the gastrocnemius and soleus that plantarflex the foot. Also known as triceps surae.

Gaucher disease: One of the most common lysosomal storage diseases with a deficiency of the enzyme glucocerebrosidase (β-glucosidase). The protein glucocerebroside accumulates, which results in hepatosplenomegaly, osteoporosis, and avascular necrosis of the distal femur.

genetic: Pertaining to reproduction or to birth of origin; hereditary traits.

genicular vessels: The vascular supply to the knee. The medial and lateral superior and inferior genicular arteries come off the popliteal artery, and the middle genicular artery comes off of the femoral artery.

genu: The knee, or the joint between the distal femur and proximal tibia.

Gerdy tubercle: A bony prominence on the lateral side of the tibia that serves as the attachment for the iliotibial band.

giant cell tumor: A benign tumor of the bone characterized by large multinucleated cells found in the epiphysis of bones. Also known as osteoclastoma.

gigantism: A medical condition in which a portion or the entire body is enlarged. May be associated with a pituitary tumor or Klippel-Trénaunay-Weber syndrome.

gigli saw: A flexible saw consisting of a wire with teeth used to cut through bone.

Girdlestone procedure: A surgical procedure where the femoral head and neck are removed but the muscles are preserved, which allows the patient to ambulate. Often performed in the setting of infection, tumor, or failed total hip arthroplasty.

glenohumeral joint: The shoulder joint, or the articulation between the lateral scapula (glenoid) and humerus.

glenolabral articular disruption (GLAD) lesion: A tear of the anteroinferior labrum and lesion of the anteroinferior articular cartilage of the glenoid due to glenohumeral impaction.

glomus tumor: A benign vascular growth at the end of fingers or toes that is small and tender.

glucosamine: An amino derivative of glucose that is a component of articular cartilage. Most commonly found in the forms of glucosamine sulfate and glucosamine hydrochloride and available as an over-the-counter nutritional supplement thought to protect cartilage.

gluteus maximus: A muscle that extends and externally rotates the hip. It originates from the ilium and dorsal sacrum and inserts into the gluteal tuberosity of the femur and the iliotibial band.

gluteus medius: A muscle that is an abductor of the hip. It originates from the ilium and inserts on the greater trochanter.

gluteus minimus: A muscle that is an abductor of the hip. It originates from the ilium and inserts on the anterior greater trochanter.

glycoprotein: A chemical composed of a protein with a conjugated carbohydrate.

golfer's elbow: Medial epicondylitis, or inflammation of the tendinous junction of the flexor carpi radialis and/or pronator teres as it arises from the medial epicondyle of the humerus.

goniometer: Instrument for measuring the range of motion at a joint.

gouge: A surgical instrument with a curved cutting end used to remove bone (eg, removal of bone when taking iliac crest bone graft).

gout: A painful metabolic disease in which crystals are deposited within a joint; often characterized by inflammation in the great toes and/or knees, along with tophi formation.

Gowers' sign: A physical exam finding where a patient uses the upper extremities to push the body into an erect position. Often found in patients with Duchenne muscular dystrophy, may also be found in congenital myopathy and spinal muscular atrophy.

gracilis: A muscle that adducts and flexes the thigh. It originates from the body of inferior pubic rami and inserts in the pes aserinus.

grade: A histological measurement of tumor severity based on the amount of dedifferentiation present. Grade 1 tumors are low-grade and well-differentiated tumors. Higher grades of tumors are poorly differentiated or undifferentiated.

graft: The replacement of a defect in the body with a portion of suitable material, either organic or inorganic.

granulation: The formation of a mass of tiny red granules of newly formed capillaries, as on the surface of a wound that is healing.

granulocyte: Any cell containing granules, especially a granular leukocyte. A heterogeneous class of leukocytes characterized by a multilobed nucleus and intracellular granules. Granulocytes include neutrophils, eosinophils, basophils, and mast cells.

Grashey view: A technique to capture radiographs of the glenohumeral joint. The patient's arm is abducted 90 degrees and the beam is directed in a 30-degree lateral oblique projection.

grasp dynamometer: Instrument used to measure the strength of a person's grip.

gray matter: Area of the central nervous system that contains the cell bodies.

greater trochanter: A bony prominence on the proximal and lateral femur where the abductors of the hip attach (gluteus medius and gluteus minimus).

greater trochanteric osteotomy: A cut in the bone to remove the greater trochanter on the femur in order to gain access to the hip joint. May be repaired with wires or a claw.

greenstick fracture: An incomplete fracture of bone in children in which one cortex is disrupted but the other cortex is not.

Grevlich-Pyle atlas: An atlas used to estimate a child's bone age based on tables and radiographic images of the wrist and hand from infancy to the end of growth.

Grice procedure: A surgical procedure used to treat congenital vertical talus by performing an extra-articular arthrodesis in children where bone graft is placed into the subtalar joint.

groin flap: A region of skin, subcutaneous tissue, and vessels (superficial circumflex iliac, superficial inferior epigastric) from the groin that may be removed as a free flap and reattached to another site or used as a pedicled flap.

growth arrest: An interruption of growth at the epiphyseal plate due to injury, infection, or surgical intervention. May result in overall shortening or angular deformity if only a portion of the epiphysis is arrested.

growth factors: Biological molecules endogenous to the body that stimulate tissue growth and repair.

growth plate: The region of cartilage between the epiphysis and metaphysis where growth occurs in bone.

guide: An instrument used to steer another instrument in a certain direction.

Guillain-Barré syndrome (acute idiopathic polyneuritis): An acute inflammatory demyelinating polyneuropathy in which the body's own immune system attacks the peripheral nervous system, which results in progressive paralysis.

guillotine amputation: Removal of an extremity in which the amputation is performed at the same level for all anatomic structures and the wound is left open.

gunstock deformity: An upper extremity deformity in which the elbow is in varus and the forearm deviates medially. Also known as cubitus varus.

Gustilo and Anderson classification: The primary classification for open fractures. Grade I: less than 1 cm; grade II: greater than 1 cm; grade IIIa: extensive damage to soft tissues with adequate soft tissue coverage; grade IIIb: extensive soft tissue damage requiring flap coverage; and grade IIIc: extensive soft tissue damage requiring vascular repair (*see* Appendix 15).

Guyon canal: A tunnel between the pisiform and hamate bones that contains the ulnar artery and nerve. May be a site of compression for the ulnar nerve.

H

Haglund deformity: A painful bony enlargement on the posterior portion of the heel, often due to excessive contact friction from shoes.

hairline fracture: A nondisplaced fracture that appears as a thin line on x-ray, resembling the thickness of hair.

half-life: (1) Measurement of the amount of time required for 50% of a drug to be eliminated from the body. (2) The time in which the radioactivity originally associated with an isotope will be reduced by one half through radioactive decay.

hallux: The first or big toe.

hallux adductus: Deviation of the first toe toward the midline.

hallux valgus: Deviation of the first toe away from the midline with an enlargement of the first metatarsophalangeal joint at the head of the first metatarsal. *Synonym*: Bunion.

halo: A ring with 4 pins (adult) or 8 pins (child) that are fixed to the skull in order to maintain the alignment or stability of the cervical spine following surgery or trauma. May be attached to a body vest for stability (*see* Appendix 18).

halo traction: Using the halo device to pull traction on the cervical spine in order to prevent a segment from dislocating.

hamartoma: A benign growth of normal tissue in an abnormal location. In orthopedics, cartilage may grow in the chest wall, and fibrous tissue may grow in the upper arm or shoulder of children under 2 years old.

hammer toe: A fixed or flexible toe deformity in which the proximal interphalangeal joint is flexed and the metatarsophalangeal joint is extended. For the first toe, the interphalangeal joint is flexed and the metatarsophalangeal joint is extended. May be a result of wearing shoes with small toe boxes. *Synonym*: Mallet toe.

Chen AF, ed.
*Quick Reference Dictionary
for Orthopedics (pp 75-83).*

Hand-Schüller-Christian disease: An aggressive form of Langerhans cell histiocytosis that is multifocal, involving bone, the hypothalamus, or pituitary stalk. Patients present with skull defects, exophthalmos (eye protrusion), and diabetes insipidus.

hanging arm cast: A treatment for humeral shaft fractures in which a cast is applied from the upper arm to the wrist and is suspended by a string or sling looped around the neck.

hangman fracture: A traumatic spondylolisthesis of the axis (second cervical vertebrae) where a fracture occurs through the pars interarticularis due to a hyperextension and distraction injury to the neck.

Hardinge approach: A direct lateral or transgluteal surgical approach to the hip.

Harrington rod: A solid steel rod used in spine surgery to hold the vertebrae aligned, used in scoliosis surgery and in instrumented fusion.

Harris hip score (HHS): A standardized questionnaire to assess the outcome of hip surgeries, by assessing radiographs, physical exam findings, and subjective pain.

Harris line: A line seen on x-ray where growth is arrested in a growing child in the epiphyses of long bones, normally following injury or a metabolic disturbance.

Haversian canals: Canals within the bone that carry blood vessels to provide nutrients to bone.

Hawkins classification: A fracture classification system for talar neck fractures (*see* Appendix 15).

Hawkins sign: Appearance of decreased subchondral bone density that is evidence of revascularization of the talar body at 6 to 8 weeks after talar injury. This sign suggests that the bone segment has adequate circulation and that normal healing is occurring.

Hawkins test: A physical exam maneuver to test supraspinatus tendon impingement. The shoulder is brought to 90 degrees of forward flexion and the arm is internally rotated; a positive Hawkins test is when pain is elicited with this maneuver.

Hawthorne effect: Research error due to the response of participants from being observed by researchers.

head-splitting fracture: A fracture of the head of the humerus or the femur that splits the head into 2 more pieces.

healing: The method by which the body repairs itself after injury.

health maintenance organization (HMO): Prepaid organized health care delivery system. Most noted for providing insurance care only within select group of clinical participants, different than a preferred provider organization (PPO).

Heberden nodules: Small growths of bone (osteophytes) at the distal interphalangeal joints often seen in osteoarthritis.

heel: The hind part of the foot.

heel cord: The tendon that attaches the gastrocsoleus to the calcaneus. *Synonym*: Achilles tendon.

heel spur: A bony protrusion from the posterior inferior calcaneus where the plantar fascia attaches or at the attachment of the Achilles tendon.

hemangioma: A benign tumor composed of small blood vessels.

hemarthrosis: Blood in the joint, due to injury or postsurgical collection of blood.

hematocrit (Hct): The volume percentage of erythrocytes in whole blood. Normal values range from 40% to 54% for males and 36% to 48% for females.

hematoma: Localized collection of blood in an organ or within tissue.

hematomyelia: Blood in the spinal cord.

hemiarthroplasty: Replacing one half of a joint with a metal prosthesis, such as the humeral head in the shoulder and the femoral head in the hip.

hemimelia: Incomplete formation or shortening of the lower segments of an extremity (forearm for the upper extremity; fibula for the lower extremity).

hemimelica: Development of osteochondromas often involving multiple bones on one limb. May be localized (one epiphysis), classic (many epiphyses on one limb), or generalized (many epiphyses on multiple limbs). Also known as Trevor disease, dysplasia epiphysealis, and epiphyseal osteochondroma.

hemiparesis: Weakness of the left or right side of the body.

hemipelvectomy: Surgical removal of the iliac wing and the remainder of the leg, often for tumor. May be external or internal. *Synonym*: Hindquarter amputation.

hemiplegia: Condition in which half of the body is paralyzed due to anoxia during birth, an aneurysm or cerebral vascular accident, or trauma.

hemivertebrae: A congenital anomaly in which only a portion of the vertebrae is formed, which leads to angular abnormalities in the vertebral columns.

hemoglobin (Hgb): The oxygen-carrying pigment of the erythrocytes formed by the developing erythrocyte in bone marrow. Normal values range from 14 to 18 g/dL for males and 12 to 16 g/dL for females.

hemolysis: The liberation of hemoglobin. The separation of the hemoglobin from the corpuscles and its appearance in the fluid in which the corpuscles are suspended.

hemophilia: Sex-linked recessive disease that results from the deficiency of factor clotting activity. Patients may present with recurrent knee hemarthroses from minimal trauma.

hemorrhage: The escape of large quantities of blood from a blood vessel; heavy bleeding.

hemovac (HV): A portable wound suction device that can hold up to 500 mL of fluid placed in surgical sites to facilitate drainage.

Henry approach: A surgical approach through the dorsal part of the forearm that utilizes the interval between the brachioradialis and the pronator teres proximally and the flexor carpi ulnaris distally. Often used to fix radial shaft fractures.

hereditary: The genetic transmission of a particular quality or trait from parent to offspring.

hereditary motor sensory neuropathy (HMSN): A syndrome in which there is progressive demyelination of the peripheral nerves that results in muscle weakness, sensory changes, and extremity deformities (cavovarus feet and claw hands).

hereditary multiple exostosis: An autosomal dominant condition in which patients form multiple benign osteochondromas, or cartilage-capped bony growths, especially around the metaphyses of long bones. May possibly become malignant and transform to chondrosarcomas.

hernia: The protrusion of all or part of an organ through a tear in the wall of the surrounding structure, such as the protrusion of part of the gastrointestinal tract through the abdominal muscles.

herniated vertebral disc: Weakness in the annulus allows the nucleus pulposus to protrude, which may press against spinal nerve roots, resulting in radicular symptoms, or against the spinal cord, resulting in myelopathy.

heroin: Highly addictive narcotic from the opium family.

herpetic whitlow: *Herpes simplex* virus (HSV) infection on a finger. HSV-1 often affects health care workers who come in contact with the mouth (eg, dentists). HSV-2 is found in the genitals.

heterotopic ossification (HO): Abnormal formation of bone from muscle. Often due to trauma, surgical procedures, comas, or high calcium concentration in blood. May lead to joint stiffness. *Synonym*: Myositis ossificans.

hex screw: A screw with a hexagonal head.

Hibbs retractor: A handheld double-ended retractor with a 90-degree bend to retract a deep wound.

Hill-Sachs lesion: A bony defect in the posterosuperior humeral head found in dislocations of the shoulder.

hindfoot: The posterior portion of the foot, including the calcaneus and talus.

hindquarter amputation: Removal of the iliac wing and entire leg. *Synonym*: Hemipelvectomy.

hinged elbow brace: A dynamic brace with adjustable ranges of motion that can be used to immobilize the elbow after a fracture or surgery. Also known as an elbow range of motion brace (*see* Appendix 18).

hinged knee brace: A dynamic brace with adjustable ranges of motion that can be used to immobilize the knee after a fracture or surgery. Also known as a postoperative knee orthosis or a Bledsoe knee brace (*see* Appendix 18).

hip: The femur and acetabular articulation.

hip disarticulation: An amputation through the hip joint with removal of the femoral head.

hip–knee–ankle–foot orthosis (HKAFO): A device to control all lower extremity segments. May be used after hip dislocations to prevent adduction and may be used after acetabular surgery to limit abduction and flexion (*see* Appendix 18).

hip spica cast: A cast that immobilizes the hip and the thigh for a femur fracture in a young child, where the hips and knees are flexed and the legs are abducted. The cast extends from the nipple line to the legs and may end above the knees or ankles. A bar may be placed between the legs to keep the legs abducted and immobilized (*see* Appendix 17).

hip spica dressing: A soft compressive dressing wrapped around the hip and the waist to compress a hip wound (*see* Appendix 17).

histiocyte: A mononuclear phagocytic macrophage found in connective tissue.

histiocytoma: A tumor composed of histiocytes surrounded by fibrous tissue.

histiocytosis X: An older term for Langerhans cell histiocytosis, which is a collection of epidermal dendritic cells (Langerhans cells) that migrate from the skin to the lymph nodes. The disease may be unifocal, multifocal unisystem, or multifocal multisystem.

Hoffa fragment: The fragment of bone from the posterior distal femoral condyle that results from a vertical fracture in the distal femoral condyle.

Hohmann retractor: A surgical device with a sharp or blunt end used to hold soft tissue out of the operative field.

Homans' sign: Pain in the posterior compartment of the leg when the ankle is slowly dorsiflexed, which may be indicative of a deep vein thrombosis.

homogeneity of variance: The statistical assumption that the variability within each of the sample groups should be fairly similar.

hook of the hamate: A bony structure off of the volar, inferior, and ulnar side of the hamate that is curved and resembles a hook. Multiple attachments occur there, including the transverse carpal ligament, the flexor carpi ulnaris, the flexor digiti minimi brevis, and the opponens digiti minimi.

hormone: A chemical substance produced in the body that has a specific effect on the activity of a certain organ; applied to substances secreted by endocrine glands and transported in the blood stream to the target organ on which their effect is produced.

housemaid knee: Inflammation of the bursa anterior to the patella, often after direct or chronic trauma, such as being on one's knees as a housemaid. *Synonym*: Prepatellar bursitis.

humeral head: The proximal end of the humerus that articulates with the glenoid to form the shoulder joint.

humerus: Long bone of the upper arm.

humpback: Spine kyphosis that results in a prominence of the upper back.

Humphrey ligament: The anterior meniscofemoral ligament, or the ligament that connects the posterior horn of the lateral meniscus to the medial femoral condyle.

Hunter canal: A tunnel made of aponeuroses in the thigh that contains the femoral artery and vein, which lies between the anterior and medial compartments.

Hunter syndrome: One of the mucopolysaccharidoses (type II) that is X-linked recessive, in which there is a deficiency of iduronate-2-sulfate that results in the build-up of heparan sulfate and dermatan sulfate. Patients present with mental retardation. Less severe than Hurler syndrome.

Huntington chorea: An autosomal dominant condition caused by a mutation of the Huntington gene that results in progressive loss of the central nervous system and presents as jerky and irregular movements.

Hurler syndrome: One of the mucopolysaccharidoses (type I) that is autosomal recessive, in which there is a deficiency of iduronidase that results in the buildup of heparan sulfate and dermatan sulfate. Patients may present with scoliosis, joint contractures, mental retardation, macroglossia, corneal clouding, and hepatosplenomegaly.

hyaline cartilage: Smooth and resilient cartilage at the end of long bones that articulate, including the humerus, glenoid, femur, and tibia. Mostly composed of type II collagen. Also found in the respiratory tract and immature skeleton.

hyaluronic acid (hyaluronan): An anionic, nonsulfated glycosaminoglycan that is a component of the extracellular matrix. It is the main constituent of synovial fluid and surrounds chondrocytes in articular cartilage. Because it is a highly negatively charged particle, it attracts water and provides lubrication of cells especially under compressive forces.

hybrid total joint replacement: A joint replacement (hip or knee) in which a combination of cemented and cementless techniques are used.

hydrocephalus: A pathological condition in which there is excess buildup of cerebrospinal fluid in the brain. May be due to obstructed outflow or decreased resorption.

hydroxyapatite (HA): A substance used as a coating for some orthopedic implants that most resembles bone and is composed of calcium and phosphorus. May facilitate bone ongrowth or ingrowth, depending on the formulation used.

hyperalgesia: Increased feeling of pain.

hyperemia: Physiological increase in blood flow to an active tissue.

hyperesthesia: Increased sensitivity to touch or other stimulation.

hyperextension: The ability of a joint to be extended beyond the normal range of motion.

hyperlordosis: Excessive lordotic curvature of the spine. *Synonym*: Swayback.

hyperostosis: An abnormal thickening of bone, such as seen in the spine for diffuse idiopathic skeletal hyperostosis (DISH).

hyperparathyroidism: A pathological condition in which an excess amount of parathyroid causes increased calcium and decreased phosphorus, which results in calcium loss from bones and increased kidney stones. A common method of remembering the symptoms of hyperparathyroidism is "Stones, bones, groans, and psychological overtones."

hyperplasia: Increased replication of one cell type that can enlarge an organ or tissue.

hyperreflexia: An overactive reflex response, often a sign of upper motor neuron damage.

hypertonia: Increased muscle tone due to spasticity.

hypertrophy: Enlargement of a portion of the body, including muscles, organs, or nerves.

hyponychium: The epithelium below the nail plate at the distal end of the nail before the skin of the fingertip. Forms a seal that protects the nail bed.

hypoplasia: Incomplete development of an organ or tissue.

hypothenar eminence: The region of the hand on the ulnar and palmar side that contains the short flexors of the small finger, including the abductor digiti minimi, flexor digiti minimi brevis, and opponens digiti minimi.

hypotonia: Decreased muscle tone.

hypotonic cerebral palsy: A type of cerebral palsy in which damage to the nervous system results in muscles with little or no tone.

hypoxia: Any state in which an inadequate amount of oxygen is available to the tissues; may be due to an obstruction of oxygen delivery or the deficiency of oxygen in the blood.

iatrogenic: An adverse condition caused by medical diagnosis or treatment.

ibuprofen: A type of nonsteroidal anti-inflammatory drug (NSAID) that inhibits both cycloogenase (COX)-1 and COX-2, producing analgesic effects as well as antiplatelet effects. Also known as iso-butyl-propanoic-phenolic acid.

Ideberg and Goss classification: A fracture classification system for glenoid fractures (*see* Appendix 15).

idiopathic: Designating a disease whose cause is unknown or uncertain.

iliac: The ilium, or the large wing of bone that forms the lateral wall of the pelvis.

iliac crest bone graft: Bone taken from the anterior or posterior iliac crest; may be autograft (often taken during spine surgery or trauma nonunion surgery) or allograft.

iliac oblique view: One of the views of the acetabulum that is a part of the Judet views. The patient is placed supine with the uninvolved side rotated anteriorly approximately 45 degrees with the beam aimed vertically at the involved hip. This view shows the posterior column of the acetabulum (ilioischial line) and the anterior wall.

iliacus: A muscle that flexes the hip. It originates from the iliac fossa and inserts into the lesser trochanter.

iliofemoral flap: A surgical technique in which the subcutaneous tissues, vessels (superficial circumflex iliac, superficial inferior epigastric), and skin are removed and reattached to another site. Also known as a groin flap.

iliopectineal bursa: A fluid-filled sac that occurs where the iliopsoas muscle and tendon contact the anterior brim of the pelvis (iliopectineal eminence).

Chen AF, ed.
Quick Reference Dictionary for Orthopedics (pp 84-91).
© 2012 Taylor & Francis Group

iliopectineal eminence: The bony ridge that is the union of the ilium and pubis that is medial to the anterior inferior iliac spine; location where the iliacus and psoas muscle pass over the pelvic brim. Also known as the iliopubic eminence.

iliopectineal line: A line seen on an anterioposterior (AP) radiograph of the pelvis that denotes the anterior column of the acetabulum. Also known as the iliopubic line.

iliopsoas: The confluence of the iliacus and psoas major muscles that flex the hip. The origin of these muscles is on the lumbar vertebrae and they insert into the lesser trochanter of the femur.

iliotibial band (ITB): The tendon of the tensor fascia lata muscle that inserts into Gerdy's tubercle on the tibia, which is used to abduct and flex the hip.

iliotibial band syndrome: A condition in which the iliotibial band rubs against the lateral femoral condyle and the friction produced causes pain. This condition is especially common in runners and may be treated by stretching (eg, foam rolling).

Ilizarov external fixator: An elaborate external fixator that uses multiple pins and wires that attach to circular rings to stabilize communited fractures and correct angular or length deformities.

imbrication: The surgical technique of overlapping tissue to increase strength and/or shorten its length.

immunoglobulin (Ig): Glycoproteins found in blood and other body fluids that may exert antibody activity. All antibodies are Ig molecules, but not all Ig exhibits antibiotic activity.

immunosuppression: A decrease in responsiveness of the immune system with an imbalance of the antigen–antibody relationship.

impacted fracture: A fracture pattern where bone fragments are wedged into one another due to the force of the injury.

impingement: To trap and compress. Often used to describe shoulder impingement or spinal nerve root impingement.

implant: Any graft or material (prosthesis, plate, screws, etc) that are placed in the body during a surgical procedure.

incidence: During a specified time period, the number of new cases of a certain illness or injury in a population. It is demonstrated as the number of new cases divided by the total number of people at risk.

incise: To cut into the body.

incision: The entrance point of a surgical procedure and the cut created from a surgical procedure.

inclusion cyst: An abnormal epithelium-lined sac in the body that contains gas, liquid, or a semisolid material.

incontinence: Inability to control excretory functions. May be present in the setting of spinal cord injury with loss of bowel and bladder habit.

indomethacin: A type of nonsteroidal anti-inflammatory drug (NSAID) that inhibits cyclooxygenase (COX)-1 and COX-2, as well as the motility of polymorphonuclear leukocytes. Indomethacin is used for analgesia and is used to treat gout in the acute phases.

induration: Abnormal firmness of tissue with a definite margin.

infantile fibromatosis: Proliferation of benign fibrous tissue in infants composed of fibroblasts and collagen, where the cells have round and small intracytoplasmic inclusions.

infantile spinal muscular dystrophy: An autosomal recessive condition that presents as muscle weakness and atrophy in infants, which makes it difficult to meet developmental milestones. Also known as Werdnig-Hoffman disease.

infarct: An area of coagulation necrosis in a tissue due to local anemia resulting from obstruction of circulation to the area.

infection: The state of being infected, especially by the presence in the body of bacteria, protozoa, viruses, or other parasites.

inference: Possible result or conclusion that could be deduced from evaluating data.

inferential (predictive) statistics: Utilizing the measurements from the sample to anticipate characteristics of the population.

inferior: In anatomical position, located below. *Synonym:* Caudal.

inferior gemellus: A muscle that is a short external rotator of the hip. It originates from the ischial tuberosity and inserts in the medial greater trochanter.

inferior vena cava (IVC) filter: A filter placed into the inferior vena cava to prevent deep vein thrombosis from entering the pulmonary vasculature.

inflammation: The condition into which tissues enter as a reaction to injury, including signs of pain (dolor), heat (calor), redness (rubor), and swelling (tumor).

informed consent: Requirement that the patient giving consent must be given adequate information about the benefits and risks of planned treatments, intervention, or research before he or she agrees to the procedures.

infrapatellar: The region below the patella.

infraspinatus: One of the rotator cuff muscles that externally rotates the arm. It originates in the infraspinatus fossa of the scapula and inserts into the greater tuberosity.

ingrown toenail: A condition in which soft tissue grows over a toenail, which leads to localized inflammation and pain, and may become infected. Often due to repetitive trauma to the region, abnormal foot structure, tight shoes, athlete's foot (fungal infections), and improper nail trimming.

inhibition: Arrest or restraint of a process.

inlay graft: A bone graft that is placed into a prefitted or precut cavity.

innominate: In a child, the bone that is the intersection of the ilium, ischium, and pubis. In the adult, these bones coalesce and form the pelvis. Also known as os coxae.

inotropic: Affecting the force or energy of muscular contractions. Either weakening or increasing the forces of muscular contraction.

inpatient: Services delivered to the patient during hospitalization.

Insall-Bernstein knee replacement (IB knee): One of the earlier total knee arthroplasty implants designed to allow the cruciates to be retained. The femur, tibia, and patella were all resurfaced, and the tibial component was only composed of one piece.

Insall-Salvati ratio: A method used to determine the position of the patella with regards to the knee. Based on a lateral x-ray of the knee, the ratio is the length of the patellar tendon divided by the length of the patella. If the ratio is less than 0.8, then the patient has a low patella (patella baja). If the ratio is greater than 1.2, then the patient has a high patella (patella alta).

insertion: Distal attachment of a muscle that exhibits most of the movement during muscular contraction. *Antonym:* Origin.

in situ: Localized site, confined to one place (eg, local tumor that has not invaded neighboring tissue).

in situ cancer: A localized cancer that remains in the tissue that it it originated from.

in situ fracture fixation: A fracture that is fixed in its original place, without manipulation.

instability: Description of a joint that has lost structural integrity and is hypermobile.

instrumentation: Tools that are used to perform surgery.

insufficiency fracture: A subgroup of stress fractures that occur in the pelvis due to physiologic stress on weakened or osteoporotic bone.

intercalary: To occur between 2 bone segments.

interclass coefficient (ICC): A statistical parameter.

intercondylar: The region between the condyles at the end of long bone.

intercostal: The region between the ribs.

interferon (IFN): A class of unrelated cytokine proteins formed when immune cells are exposed to viruses. There are 3 main classes: alpha, beta, and gamma. Pharmaceutical drugs have been manufactured to boost the host immune response and kill tumor cells.

intermetaral neuroma: A benign collection of nerve tissue in the foot, commonly in the third and fourth metatarsals. Also known as a Morton neuroma.

intermuscular: The region between muscles; often refers to a surgical plane.

internal fixation: A surgical procedure in which hardware is secured directly onto bone (eg, rods, plates, or screws) to achieve fracture fixation.

internal rotation: Turning toward the midline or turning inward.

internal tibial torsion (ITT): A condition in which the distal tibia is rotated toward the midline. It is one of the etiologies that cause intoeing.

internal validity: The cause-and-effect relationship that can be identified by the results of an experiment.

International Classification of Diseases (ICD): Disease classification system developed by the World Health Organization; codes that may be used for billing and reimbursement purposes.

International Normalized Ratio (INR): A measurement of clotting through the extrinsic clotting cascade that is calculated by dividing the prothrombin time (PT) of the test by the PT of a normal individual. For patients who are anticoagulated after orthopedic procedures, the goal INR is often 2.0 to 3.0. Warfarin is an example of a drug that increases the INR.

internervous plane: A surgical plane between 2 muscles that have different nerve supplies that is often used for dissection.

interossei muscles: The 2 layers of small muscles between the metacarpals in the hand and the metatarsals in the foot that cause digit abduction and adduction.

interphalangeal (IP): The region between fingers and toes.

interscalene nerve block: A regional delivery of local anesthetic agent in the interscalene region (between the anterior and middle scalene muscles) that reduces pain and sensation in the arm (brachial plexus distribution).

interspinous ligament: The dense tissue that connects adjacent spinous processes of the vertebrae to stabilize the posterior.

intertrochanteric fracture: A fracture that travels between the greater and lesser trochanters in the femur. Often surgically fixed with a cephallomedullary device or dynamic hip screw (DHS).

interval data: Measurements that are assigned values so that the order and intervals between numbers are recognized.

intervertebral discs: A structure between the vertebral bodies that cushions the vertebrae and absorbs shock. They are composed of an inner nucleus pulposus (water and aggrecan) and an outer, tougher annulus fibrosus, consisting of type I collagen in concentric lamellae.

intra-articular: Within a joint.

intracapsular ankylosing: Autofusion of a joint within the capsule, often due to inflammation or infection.

intramedullary: Inside the medullary canal of the bone. May refer to guides used in arthroplasty surgery that enter the medullary canal or the position of nails to fix fractures.

intramedullary nail: A surgical implant placed within the center canal of a long bone (eg, femur, tibia, and humerus) to fix a fracture or osteotomy.

intramuscular (IM): Within the muscle or a drug administered into a muscle.

intraosseous (IO): Within the bone.

intraosseous lipoma: A benign fatty tumor within bone.

intrapelvic obturator neurectomy: Surgically cutting the obturator nerve in the pelvis for cerebral palsy patients to diminish adductor muscle spasticity.

intraspinal lesion: Any mass within the spine, either a tumor or abscess.

intravenous (IV): Situated within or administered into a vein (eg, IV drug entered through the vein).

intrinsic: Coming from or originating from within.

intrinsic muscles: The muscles within the hands and feet that work to abduct and adduct the fingers and toes.

intrinsic palsy: Paralysis of the intrinsic muscles of the hand and/or feet.

intrinsic plus position: The safe position for hand splinting, where the wrist is extended, the metacarpophalangeal (MCP) joint is flexed, and the interphalangeal joint is extended.

invaginating: An anatomic structure that folds on itself.

invasive test: A test that requires penetration of the body (eg, arteriogram).

inversion: Turning inward.

inversion ankle stress test: A physical exam in which the ankle is maximally turned inwards to assess the stability of the ankle ligaments. Often done under x-ray fluoroscopy to assess the stability of ankle, especially after fracture fixation. Also known as a talar tilt test.

in vitro: An experiment conducted outside of an organism (eg, cell culture).

in vivo: An experiment conducted inside an organism (eg, animals, humans).

involucrum: New bone that forms around a sequestrum, or infected dead bone, in osteomyelitis.

ipsilateral: Situated on or affecting the same side. *Antonym:* Contralateral.

irrigation: Applying fluid (often saline) to clean an area. May have antibiotics added to it.

ischemia: Reduced oxygen supply to a body organ or part. Deficiency of blood in a part due to functional constriction or actual obstruction of a blood vessel.

ischial: Refers to the ischium of the pelvis or the region between the pubis and the back of the ilium.

island pedicle graft: A graft where a small area of skin is transferred to another area with attached nerves and vascular supply.

isometric contraction: Static muscle contraction in which the muscle generates tension but does not change length.

isometry of ligaments: Maintaining the constant length of a ligament; often a goal of ligament reconstruction.

isotonic contraction: Contraction of a muscle during which the force of resistance remains constant throughout the range of motion.

J

Jackson table: A radiolucent surgical table used during fracture fixation, so that fluoroscopic images can be taken.

Jackson-Pratt (JP) drain: A flat drain placed within a surgical wound, with a bulb used to suction out excess fluid. May hold up to 100 mL of fluid.

Jefferson fracture: A burst fracture of the atlas (first cervical vertebrae), classically described as a 4-part fracture with anterior and posterior arch fractures.

jersey finger: Rupture of the flexor digitorum profundus (FDP) tendon, classically described as "getting a finger caught in a football jersey."

Jewett brace: A hyperextension trunk brace that provides a single 3-point force system via a sternal pad, a suprapubic pad, and a thoracolumbar pad that restricts forward flexion in the thoracolumbar area (*see* Appendix 18).

jig: A surgical device used during arthroplasty surgery that is placed on bone to guide cuts.

Jobst boot: An elastic stocking applied to an extremity to reduce swelling.

joint: Junction in the body where 2 or more bones articulate.

joint capsule: Any sac or membrane enclosing the junction of the bones.

joint mouse: A loose body within a joint, often composed of small pieces of cartilage or bone that have broken loose or formed within a synovial cavity.

joint replacement: A surgical procedure by which the bearing surfaces of a joint (shoulder, hip, knee, ankle, etc) are replaced with artificial components.

joint space narrowing: A reduction of joint space seen on x-ray due to cartilage wear, indicative of osteoarthritis.

Jones fracture: A fracture at the base of the fifth metatarsal (metaphyseal–diaphyseal junction) that have a higher rate of nonunion compared to other fractures.

Chen AF, ed.
*Quick Reference Dictionary
for Orthopedics (pp 92-93).*

Judet view: Two views of the pelvis taken at different angles that allow clearer visualization of the columns and walls of the acetabulum. One view is an obturator (internal) oblique and the other view is the iliac (external) oblique view.

jump distance: A term used in total hip arthroplasty pertaining to the maximum distance between the acetabulum and femoral head before the hip dislocates.

jumper knee: Patella tendon irritation secondary to overuse of the tendon.

juvenile aponeurotic fibroma: Benign calcifying tumors commonly found within the aponeuroses of the hand and feet of children and adolescents.

juvenile kyphosis: A form of spinal skeletal deformity in which 3 consecutive vertebrae are wedged and there are growth plate irregularities that results in kyphosis. *Synonym*: Scheuermann disease.

juvenile rheumatoid arthritis (JRA): A common form of autoimmune arthritis found in children. There are different categories of JRA: (1) polyarticular JRA, which involves many joints (large and small); (2) pauciarticular JRA, which involves a few joints (hips, knees, or ankles); and (3) systemic JRA, which presents with pain, fevers, and rashes.

juxtacortical chondroma: A chondroma beneath the periosteum and under the cortex.

Keller procedure: A surgical procedure to treat hallux valgus (bunion) where a portion of the proximal phalanx of the first toe is removed to correct alignment.

keloid: A benign overgrowth of scar tissue or skin after surgery or injury, often found in people with darker skin.

keratoma: A callus of keratin tissue.

KERLIX dressing: (Covidien, Mansfield, Massachusetts) A trademarked name of a type of dressing made of elasticized cotton used to hold dressings in place by wrapping it around extremities or used to pack wounds.

Kerrison rongeur: A surgical instrument that bites bone in small amounts, often used in the spine.

Ketorolac: A type of nonsteroidal anti-inflammatory drug (NSAID) that is available in oral and intravenous (IV) formulations that reduces prostaglandin synthesis.

key pinch: A method of pinching a small and flat object between the thumb and index finger (eg, key). If there is decreased key pinch strength, this is indicative of intrinsic muscle weakness in the hand and ulnar nerve palsy.

Kienböck disease: Loss of blood supply (avascular necrosis) to the lunate (one of the carpal bones).

kinematics: An area of kinesiology concerned with measuring, describing, and recording motions.

kinetic chain: A complex motor system formed by a series of joints. **Open:** series of joints in which the distal one is free. **Closed:** series of joints in which the distal one meets sufficient external resistance to prohibit or restrain its free motion.

kinetics: The study of motion.

Kirner deformity: A sporadic deformity of the small finger in which the distal phalanx is flexed and deviates radially; most commonly found in teenage girls.

Chen AF, ed.
*Quick Reference Dictionary
for Orthopedics (pp 94-96).*
© 2013 Tudor & Francis Group

Kirschner wire (K-wire): A steel wire of various sizes that may be threaded or smooth used to stabilize fractures or joints.

Kling dressing: (Johnson & Johnson, New Brunswick, New Jersey) The trademark name of a type of cotton dressing that is used to hold bandages and wrap extremities.

Klippel-Feil syndrome: A congenital condition in which there is a failure of segmentation of the cervical vertebrae at 3 to 8 weeks gestation, which results in fused cervical segments (most commonly C2 to 3). Patients present with short necks, low hairlines, and decreased cervical motion. May be associated with Sprengel's deformity or elevation of the scapula.

Klippel-Trénaunay-Weber syndrome: A congenital condition in which the blood and lymphatic vessels fail to properly form. Patients present with port wine stains (nevus flammeus), venous malformations (varicose veins) or lymphatic malformation, and soft tissue hypertrophy. *Synonyms*: Angioosteohypertrophy syndrome, hemangiectatic hypertrophy.

knee: A hinged joint formed by the distal femur and proximal tibia. *Synonym*: Genu.

kneecap: A common name for the patella, or the bone in the anterior knee that contributes to the extensor mechanism.

knee disarticulation: An amputation through the knee joint. Often performed as a temporizing surgery because it is a relatively quick operation that does not require bone cuts and decreases blood loss.

knock knees: A common name for valgus knees, or knees that are pointed toward the midline with the feet wide apart. *Synonyms:* Genu valgum, tibia valga.

knuckles: A common name for the metacarpophalangeal joints in the hand.

Kocher clamp: A surgical instrument with serrated surfaces and pointed teeth that is used clamp tissue.

Kocher-Langenbeck approach: A posterior surgical approach to the hip and the acetabulum that is often used for acetabular fracture fixation.

Kohler disease: Avascular necrosis or osteochondrosis of the patella or navicular bone in the foot.

Kohler line: The ilioischial line seen on an anteroposterior (AP) pelvis x-ray.

Krabbe disease: An autosomal recessive infantile condition defined by degeneration of the myelin sheath caused by a deficiency of galactocerebrosidase. This results in rapid deterioration of the central nervous system and often death by age 2. Also known as globoid cell leukodystrophy and diffuse infantile familial sclerosis.

KT-1000: (MEDmetric Corporation, San Diego, California) The trademark name of an instrument used to measure the amount of anterior translation of the tibia relative to the femur with regard to measuring the competency of the anterior and posterior cruciate ligaments.

Kugelberg-Welander syndrome: An autosomal recessive form of spinal muscular atrophy caused by a degeneration of motor neurons in the ventral horn of the spinal cord that typically appears late in the first decade of life. Also known as a spinal muscular atrophy type III.

kyphoplasty: A surgical method for treating vertebral fractures in which a needle is percutaneously inserted into a fractured vertebra, a small balloon is inserted to inflate the collapsed vertebral body, and bone cement or filler is injected to stabilize the fracture and strengthen the weakened bone. This restores the height and stability of the vertebral bone. This contrasts with vertebroplasty, in which a balloon is not used.

kyphoscoliosis: Posterior and lateral curvature of the spine, as seen in vertebral osteochondrosis (Scheuermann disease).

kyphosis: Abnormal anteroposterior curvature of the thoracic spine. Also known as hunchback or roundback.

labrum: A lip of fibrocartilage that lines the articular surface of certain bones, including the glenoid and acetabulum. It serves to deepen the socket and aids in maintaining joint stability.

Lachman test: A physical exam test for anterior cruciate ligament (ACL) stability in which the patient is placed supine on the examining table, the knee is flexed to 30 degrees, one hand is placed behind the patient's tibia and the other hand is used to stabilize the thigh, and an anterior stress is placed on the tibia. An anterior translation of greater than 10 mm, usually without a firm endpoint, indicates that there is a tear in the ACL.

lacuna: A small cavity in bone or cartilage that contains osteocytes and chondrocytes, respectively.

lag screw: A screw with a smooth segment adjacent to the head and threads distally. When tightened, the screw threads engage in the far cortex and bring the near cortex to it in order to compress the fracture site.

lamellar bone: Bone that has collagen aligned into parallel sheets to give the bone more strength than woven bone.

lamina: The posterior arch of each vertebra that overlies the spinal cord and serves as an attachment for the back muscles.

laminar flow: A type of air flow in which there is a continuous flow of highly filtered air that is recirculated under positive pressure to remove contaminated air from the surgical field.

laminectomy: Surgical excision of the posterior arch of the vertebrae to relieve pressure from the spinal cord or nerve roots.

laminotomy: Surgical removal of a portion of the lamina to gain access to and decompress the spinal cord or nerve root.

Langerhans cell histiocytosis (LCH): A group of disorders characterized by the proliferation of epidermal dendritic cells (Langerhans cells) that migrate from the skin to the lymph nodes. The disease may be unifocal, multifocal unisystem, or multifocal multisystem.

Langerhans cells: An immature dendritic cell of the epidermis that contains large granules.

Langerhans granules: Granules within Langerhans cells that are racket-shaped and membrane bound. *Synonym:* Birbeck granules.

Langer's lines: Lines in the skin that parallel joint creases; often used for surgical incisions to minimize scar formation.

lapidus procedure: A surgical procedure to correct bunions in which the first metatarsal bone is fused to the medial cuneiform bone.

Larsen's syndrome: An autosomal dominant disorder characterized by ligamentous laxity resulting in multiple joint dislocations, flattening of the face, and widely spaced eyes. It is due to a defect in growth hormone (GH) receptors that results in high levels of GH and low levels of insulin-like growth factor-1 (IGF-1).

lateral: Anatomic position located away from the midline of the body.

lateral decubitus: A surgical position where the patient is placed on their side. The patient may be held up with a pegboard, a Montreal positioner, or a beanbag.

lateralizing osteotomy of the calcaneus: A surgical procedure to treat varus deformity of the hindfoot, in which an axial cut is made through the calcaneus, and the calcaneus is slid laterally and surgically fixed.

Lauge-Hansen classification: A fracture classification system based on the stress placed on the ankle during injury (pronation, supination, abduction, adduction, and eversion) (*see* Appendix 15).

Leadbetter maneuver: A method of relocating a posteriorly dislocated hip in which the hip is flexed and internally rotated to disengage the femoral head and then traction is applied and the hip is abducted and extended.

Lederhosen disease: Scarring of the plantar fascia that produces painful nodules along the plantar surface of the feet. *Synonym*: Plantar fibromatosis.

leg: The area containing the anatomical structures between the knee and the ankle.

Legg-Calvé-Perthes (LCP) disease: Spontaneous avascular necrosis of the capital femoral epiphysis in children that leads to flattening and collapse of the femoral head. Also known as Perthes disease, coxa plana, and osteochondritis deformans juvenilis.

leg length discrepancy (LLD): Asymmetrical length of the lower extremities when one is compared to the other.

leiomyosarcoma: A rare malignant tumor of smooth muscles. Surgical treatment often entails wide resection.

length of stay (LOS): The duration of hospitalization, usually expressed in days.

lesser trochanter: A small bony prominence on the proximal posteromedial portion of the femur where the iliopsoas attaches.

Letournel classification: A fracture classification system for the acetabulum (*see* Appendix 15).

Letterer-Siwe disease: The most severe form of Langerhans cell histiocytosis, which is multifocal and multisystem (disseminated). Patients present with skin lesions that look like seborrheic dermatitis, hepatosplenomegaly (enlarged liver and spleen), and progressive anemia.

leukocyte: White blood cell in the immune system that defends the body from infection and foreign material.

leukocyte esterase: A test for the enzyme esterase that is released by white blood cells that is indicative of infection. Used to detect urinary tract infections and may be used to detect infections in other fluids, such as synovial fluid.

leukodystrophy: A group of hereditary disorders characterized by white matter deterioration in the central nervous system.

levator scapulae: A muscle that elevates the scapula. It originates from C1 to C4 transverse processes and inserts in the superior medial scapula.

Lhermitte sign: A sign of meningeal irritation when flexion of the neck and hip result in pain down the spine.

ligament: Fibrous thickening of an articular capsule that joins 2 articulating bones.

ligamentum flavum: The ligament that connects the facet joints in the spine that cover the dura mater and protect the spinal cord.

ligamentum mucosum: The small ligament in the knee anterior to the anterior cruciate ligament that holds the fat pad in a stable position.

ligamentum teres: The ligament that holds the femoral head to the inferior part of the acetabulum. The ligamentum teres contains blood vessels that supply the femoral head in young children.

ligation: A surgical procedure in which an anatomical channel is tied off (eg, tying off a blood vessel).

ligature: An object used to tie something tightly; in surgery, thread used to tie off blood vessels.

limb: An extremity, or an arm or a leg.

limb salvage: A surgical procedure to save an extremity affected by bone tumor, extensive trauma, or multiple previous surgeries.

linea aspera: A prominent large ridge on the posterior aspect of the femur that extends from the lesser trochanter to above the knee, where the adductors and intermuscular septum attach.

linear fracture: A break in the bone that extends along the length of the bone instead of transversely.

linear scleroderma: An autoimmune disorder in which there is an overproduction of abnormal collagen that results in hardening (sclerosis) and scarring (fibrosis) that affects the skin and subcutaneous tissue, which gives the appearance of leather.

lipid: A fat molecule that is used to compose the cell membranes of plant and animal cells.

lipid storage disease: A group of hereditary disorders of lipid metabolism that affect specific enzymes and result in diseases of varying severity.

lipofibroma: A benign tumor of muscle and fatty tissue.

lipoma: A benign tumor of fat that presents as a mobile mass that is often palpable under the skin.

liposarcoma: A malignant fatty tumor that arises from deep soft tissue.

Lisfranc amputation: An amputation through the Lisfranc joint, or removal of the foot through the tarsometatarsal joint.

Lisfranc dislocation: A traumatic dislocation of the foot at the Lisfranc joint that involves disruption of ligaments and is often associated with fractures of the surrounding bones. Noted on x-ray by the loss of alignment between the second metatarsal and the medial cuneiform bone.

Lisfranc joint: The tarsometatarsal joint, or the joint between the metatarsals and the tarsal bones (cuneiforms and cuboid). *Synonym*: Midtarsal joint.

Lister tubercle: A bony prominence on the dorsal surface of the distal end of the radius that serves as a pulley for the extensor pollicis longus (EPL).

listhesis: The translation of one surface across another, often used to describe the translation of one vertebra in relation to an adjacent vertebra.

little league elbow: Medial epicondylitis of the humerus at the elbow often caused by repetitive throwing motions.

little league shoulder: Apophysitis of the proximal humerus often caused by repetitive throwing injuries.

local anesthetic: A drug used to temporarily remove sensation in a specific part of the body that is regional (eg, digital block for a finger). A drug may be injectable or topical (applied to a surface).

locking compression plate: An orthopedic implant that is a plate with offset holes that allows fractured bones to be compressed with the application of locking screws.

locking plate: An orthopedic plate composed of titanium or stainless steel that is used for fracture fixation with threaded holes so that screws lock into the plate. By creating one construct, the implant may be less likely to fail.

locking screws: Screws with threaded heads that are fixed into plates.

locking suture: A running stitch that is looped within itself so that each stitch will not slide.

long arm cast (LAC): A cast that extends from just below the axilla to proximal to the heads of the metacarpals, with elbow flexion to 90 degrees, that is molded in the supracondylar humerus region and the interosseous membrane between the radius and the ulna (*see* Appendix 17).

long arm splint (LAS): A splint where plaster is applied to the posterior arm with the elbow at 90 degrees of flexion and is secured with an elastic bandage. May apply side slabs to improve the strength of the splint (*see* Appendix 17).

long bone: A long cylindrical bone that has growth plates on either end.

longitudinal axis: The long axis in the body (from the head to the toes).

longitudinal research: Study design in which subjects are measured prospectively over the course of time to gather data on potential trends.

long leg cast (LLC): A cast that extends from the proximal thigh to the heads of the metatarsals, with slight knee flexion and ankle dorsiflexion to 90 degrees, that is molded in the supracondylar femur region, the Achilles tendon, and arch (*see* Appendix 17).

long leg splint (LLS): A splint where plaster is applied to the posterior leg and the medial and lateral sides of the leg and secured with an elastic bandage where there is slight knee flexion and ankle dorsiflexion to 90 degrees (*see* Appendix 17).

long leg walking cast (LLWC): A long leg cast where the plantar surface of the foot is reinforced to allow the patient to ambulate.

long thoracic nerve: The nerve that originates from cervical nerves 5 through 7 that innervates the serratus anterior muscle and keeps the scapula from winging outwards.

loose body: An object within a joint that is detached and is free floating. May be referred to as a joint mouse.

lordosis: Anterior curvature of the spine. Normal in the cervical and lumbar spines.

Lou Gehrig disease: A progressive degeneration of the spinal nerves that control voluntary function that leads to muscle weakness and eventual death. Popularized by the famous New York Yankees player Lou Gehrig, who was afflicted by this disease. *Synonyms:* Amyotrophic lateral sclerosis (ALS), motor neuron disease.

low contact dynamic compression plate (LC-DCP): A plate that has indents to minimize the amount of contact with bone, with the purpose of preserving as much vascularity as possible. This orthopedic implant compresses fractures together with offset holes.

lower motor neuron (LMN): Sensory neuron found in the anterior horn cell, nerve root, or peripheral nervous system.

lower motor neuron (LMN) disease: A disease of the anterior horn cells in the spinal cord that controls motor functions to the extremities that leads to flaccid or atrophied muscles, muscle fasciculations, hyporeflexia, or paralysis.

Lowe syndrome: An autosomal recessive condition due to abnormalities in glycosaminoglycan metabolism that produces renal dysfunction, congenital eye disorders (glaucoma, cataracts), and mental retardation. Orthopedic manifestations include recurrent fractures from rickets, joint hypermobility, joint effusions, and tenosynovitis.

Ludloff approach: An anteromedial approach to the hip through the adductor longus and brevis, often used for congenital hip relocation or aspiration from the hips of pediatric patients.

Ludloff sign: A physical exam finding in which there is ecchymosis on the medial thigh and patients have difficult rising from a sitting position, secondary to trauma where the apophysis of the lesser trochanter is pulled off.

lumbago: A nonspecific term describing pain in the mid- and lower back.

lumbar: The region of the lower back proximal to the pelvis.

lumbar agenesis: A congenital anomaly in which there is an incomplete development of the lumbar spine, often associated with other abnormalities (eg, VATER association).

lumbarization: A condition in which the first sacral vertebra presents as a sixth lumbar vertebra if it does not fuse with the remaining sacral vertebrae.

lumbar puncture: A procedure in which a needle is inserted into the dura to remove cerebrospinal fluid or to inject anesthetic agents or dye.

lumbar spine: The 5 large spinal vertebrae proximal to the sacrum.

lumbosacral plexus: The exiting nerve roots from the lumbar and sacral spines that comprise the sciatic and femoral nerves.

lumbosacral transitional vertebrae (LSTV): When the last lumbar vertebra or first sacral vertebra has an elongated transverse process. Also called sacralized L5 or lumbarized S1.

lumbrical muscles: Small muscles of the hand and foot that flex at the metocarpophalangeal and metatarsophalangeal joints, respectively, and extend at the proximal and distal interphalangeal joints.

lumen: A hollow area that may be used to describe an organ or surgical instrument.

lunate: A carpal bone in the proximal row between the navicular and triquetrium that looks like a moon (lateral projection of the wrist) and articulates with the capitate and radius.

lupus: A systemic autoimmune disease in which antibody-immune complexes form (type III hypersensitivity); commonly affects joints (knees, hands, and wrists), kidneys, skin, and retinas.

Lyme disease: An inflammatory disease caused by the spirochete *Borrelia burgdorferi* carried by ticks that results in arthritis (often of the knee), cardiac, and neurological disorders.

lymphadenopathy: An abnormal enlargement of lymph nodes, often indicative of localized infection or tumor.

lymphangioma: A congenital tumor of the lymphatic system, also known as a cystic hygroma.

lymphedema: Swelling of an extremity caused by obstruction of the lymphatic vessels.

lymph nodes: A part of the immune system consisting of collections of lymphocytes along lymph vessels that serve as filters of tissue fluid; when swollen, may indicate an infection or tumor in that region.

lymphoma: A variety of malignant tumors arising from lymphoid tissue.

lyophilization of bone: A freeze-drying method for preserving a bone as a graft. Bone is frozen and then the frozen fluid portion of the bone is evaporated in a vacuum so that the ice sublimes (goes from solid to gas).

lysis: The destruction of soft tissue or bone.

lytic: Any process that results in lysis.

maceration: Softening of tissue by soaking in fluids. May occur in postoperative wounds when soaking in a bathtub.

macrodactyly: A congenital abnormality in which patients have enlarged digits.

macrophage: A phagocyte cell residing in tissues and derived from monocytes.

Madelung deformity: A congenital abnormality of the wrist in which there is a disturbance of the inferior volar growth plate of the distal radius that results in the radius growing volarly and the ulna growing dorsally. This often presents in adolescent females where the entire wrist and hand are translated volarly.

Maffucci syndrome: A condition in which multiple benign enchondromas occur in bone simultaneously with hemangiomas.

magnetic resonance imaging (MRI): A type of nonionizing radiographical imaging using magnetic fields and radio frequencies to produce an image; often used to visualize soft tissue structures (*see* Appendix 22).

Maisonneuve fracture: A fracture pattern in which the medial malleolus on the tibia is associated with a proximal fibular fracture, indicating that there is a disruption of the syndesmotic membrane between the tibia and fibula.

malignant fibrous histiocytoma (MFH): An outdated term used to describe a malignant sarcoma that arises in both soft tissue and bone composed of fibrous cells and multiple histiocytes.

malleolus: A bony prominence on the medial and lateral side of the ankle due to the distal ends of the tibia and fibula, respectively.

Chen AF, ed.
Quick Reference Dictionary for Orthopedics (pp 106-117).
© 2013 T

mallet finger: A finger where the extensor mechanism has been ruptured and patients present with flexion at the distal interphalangeal joint. Treated with a stack splint.

mallet fracture: A fracture of the distal phalanx with an extensor tendon avulsion that presents with a flexed distal interphalangeal joint. Also known as a bony mallet.

mallet toe: A condition in which the proximal interphalangeal joints in the second, third, and fourth toes are flexed and the metatarsophalangeal joint is extended. *Synonym*: Hammer toe.

malum coxae senilis: An older term used to describe the femoral head affected by osteoarthritis.

malunion: A fracture that has not healed in anatomic alignment.

manipulation under anesthesia (MUA): A surgical procedure performed to improve articular range of motion by breaking up scar tissue and mobilizing soft tissue while the patient is under anesthesia.

Mann-Whitney U test: A statistical test on rank-ordered data of the hypothesis of difference between 2 independent random samples. The independent t test is its ordinal likeness.

manubrium: The upper portion of the sternum.

march fracture: A stress fracture of one of the metatarsal bones in the foot that is caused by repetitive and prolonged activity, such as marching or running.

Marfan syndrome: An autosomal dominant connective tissue disorder in which there is a mutation in the gene that produces fibrillin-1 that results in an increase in transforming growth factor-beta (TGF-β). Patients present with abnormally long limbs, hypermobile joints, arachnodactyly, scoliosis, kyphosis, flat feet, and aortic aneurysms.

Markell shoes: Used to treat metatarsus adductus in the pediatric population where the left and right shoes are switched.

Maroteaux-Lamy syndrome: One of the mucopolysaccharidosis syndromes (type VI) in which there is a deficiency of arylsulfatase B and an accumulation of dermatan sulfate. Patients present with skeletal dysplasia, short stature, kyphosis, joint stiffness, and normal intelligence.

marrow: Spongy tissue that fills the medullary canal in the diaphysis of bones that is composed of fat in adults and blood-forming agents in young people.

marsupialization: A surgical procedure in which an incision is made into a cyst or the skin and the outer and inner edges are sutured together to form a pouch. This allows the area to continue to drain so that healing can take place from within. Named for mammals that carry their young in pouches (eg, kangaroos).

Mason classification: A fracture classification system for radial head fractures based on comminution and the amount of bone involved (*see* Appendix 15).

matrix: The microscopic substance that gives tissues or cells its structure.

Mayo classification: A fracture classification system for olecranon fractures based on the degree of displacement and comminution (*see* Appendix 15).

Mayo scissors: A blunt-tipped surgical instrument with a shorter handle-to-blade ratio used to cut sutures and less delicate tissue (fascia) closer to the surface of the skin. May be curved or straight.

McBride procedure: A series of distal soft tissue releases indicated for an incongruent metatarsophalangeal joint with mild hallux valgus deformity. Often used concomitantly with distal osteotomy procedures. Currently modified to retain the lateral sesamoid, which helps prevent hallux varus.

McCune-Albright syndrome: A genetic disease characterized by precocious puberty in females, fibrous dysplasia lesions, and multiple café au lait spots. *Synonym*: Polyostotic fibrous dysplasia.

McMurray test: A physical exam used to test for meniscal tears. The knee is flexed to 90 degrees and one hand is placed on the joint line of the knee. The other hand holds the plantar surface of the foot in external rotation (for the medial meniscus) or internal rotation (for the lateral meniscus). If there is a palpable or audible click when extending the leg, the test suggests that there is a meniscus tear.

mean: Arithmetic average. One of the measures of central tendency.

mean arterial pressure (MAP): The average arterial blood pressure during one cardiac cycle, which is the sum of one third of the systolic blood pressure and two thirds of the diastolic blood pressure. In many orthopedic surgery cases where bleeding should be minimized, the MAP can be kept low using regional hypotensive anesthesia.

meatus: Passage or opening within a body.

medial: Anatomic position located closer to the midline of the body.

medial parapatellar approach: A surgical approach to the knee in which the incision is started in the midline but the capsular incision curves to the medial side of the patella. This is the most common approach to the knee for total knee arthroplasty.

median: The value or score that most closely represents the middle of a range of scores. One of the measures of central tendency.

median nerve: One branch of the brachial plexus that provides motor function to the first and second lumbricals, opponens pollicis, abductor pollicis brevis, and flexor pollicis brevis. It provides sensory innervation to the skin of the palmar side of the thumb, index, middle, and half of the ring finger. It is the nerve that is compressed in carpal tunnel syndrome.

mediastinum: The mass of tissues and organs separating the 2 lungs, between the sternum in front and the vertebral column behind and from the thoracic inlet above to the diaphragm below. It contains the heart and its large vessels, trachea, esophagus, thymus, lymph nodes, and other structures and tissues.

Medical Research Council Scale for Muscle Strength: A grading scheme in which muscle strength is rated from 0 (no contraction) to 5 (normal muscle strength) (*see* Appendix 12).

medullary: Marrow in the center portion of an organ or bone.

Mehta angle: A radiographic measurement to determine if a curve will progress in infantile idiopathic scoliosis. The angle is measured between the apical vertebra of the curve and either rib on the side of that vertebra. If the rib vertebral angle is greater than 20 degrees, the curve is more likely to progress. *Synonym*: Rib vertebral angle (RVA).

Meige disease: A disease of familial lymphedema that causes pitting in the legs. *Synonym*: Milroy disease.

melorheostosis: A form of hyperostosis in which there is a mutation in the LEMD3 gene that leads to mesenchymal dysplasia and unilateral cortical thickening that looks like melting candle wax.

Meloxicam: A nonsteroidal anti-inflammatory drug (NSAID) that inhibits cyclooxygenase (COX) and achieves high concentrations within synovial fluid.

meningocele: One form of spina bifida in which the posterior elements of the spinal column do not unite (laminae) and the meninges protrude posteriorly. May be associated with tethered cord.

meningomyelocoele: A severe form of spina bifida in which the meninges and spinal cord protrude through the posterior elements of the spinal column. Also known as a myelomeningocele. There is often loss of neurologic function below the affected level.

meniscus: The C-shaped fibrocartilage attached to the tibia that acts as a shock absorber in the knee. There is a medial and lateral meniscus.

menisectomy: Surgical removal of a portion or the entire meniscus, including torn meniscus fragments.

Merchant view: A technique to capture radiographs of the patella in which the patient is supine on the table and the knee is flexed to 45 degrees. The beam is then directed distally from the superior patella at 30 degrees from the horizontal axis.

meta-analysis: Type of research in which previous research studies are aggregated to determine outcome trends.

metacarpophalangeal (MCP, MP) joint: The articulating joint in the hand between the head of the metacarpal bone and the proximal phalanx of the fingers or thumb.

metachromatic leukodystrophy (MLD): The most common autosomal recessive lipid storage disease where arylsulfatase A is deficient and there is an excessive buildup of sulfatides. Patients present with central nervous system deterioration and abnormal muscle movements. There are 3 forms of the disease: late infantile, juvenile, and adult.

metaphyseal chondrodysplasia: A defect in the hypertrophic and proliferative zones of the physis that leads to short stature, lumbar lordosis, and varus knees. *Synonym*: Metaphyseal dysostosis.

metaphyseal dysplasia: An autosomal recessive condition in which there is an abnormality of the bone remodeling process in the metaphysis. The metaphysis is abnormally thinned and flared. *Synonym*: Pyle disease.

metaphysis: The flared portion of long bone.

metastasis: The transfer of cancer cells or microorganisms to a distant site from a primary site, which produces a similar disease in a new location.

metatarsalgia: A general description of pain in the metatarsals, most commonly affecting the first metatarsus where the 2 sesamoid bones lie.

metatarsophalangeal (MTP) joint: The articulating joint in the foot between the head of the metatarsal bone and the proximal phalanx.

metatarus: The forefoot, which includes the 5 metatarsals and the phalanges of the toes.

metatropic dwarf: A type of dwarfism in which the severity of congenital skeletal dysplasia increases with growth. Initially, the trunk grows relative to the limbs, but with increased growth, the limbs outgrow the trunk.

methylene blue: A blue dye that has multiple uses in orthopedics. Methylene blue may be injected into a joint, and extravasation of the dye through a laceration would indicate an open joint. Methylene blue may be added to bone cement to accelerate the hardening of the cement and to discriminate between cement and bone.

methylprednisolone: A synthetic glucocorticoid drug used as an anti-inflammatory medication to treat inflammatory and allergic diseases.

Metzenbaum scissors: A surgical instrument with a longer handle-to-blade ratio used to cut delicate tissue.

Meyers and McKeever classification: A fracture classification system for tibial spine fractures (*see* Appendix 15).

micromelic dwarf: A type of dwarfism in which patients are characterized by short arms.

microwave diathermy: A treatment method of using shorter microwaves of higher frequency to heat deep tissue.

midaxillary line: A sagittal line drawn from the middle of the armpit to the iliac crest.

middle third: A term used to denote the middle portion of the bone, after it has been divided into thirds (proximal, middle, distal). Often used to describe clavicle fractures.

midsagittal plane: An anatomical plane used to divide the body into right and left halves.

midtarsal joint: The joint between the metatarsal and the cuneiforms and cuboid. *Synonym*: Lisfranc joint.

Milch classification: A fracture classification system of lateral condyle fractures in the pediatric patient population (*see* Appendix 15).

milk-alkali syndrome: A condition of excessive calcium and alkali ingestion (for peptic ulcer treatment) that results in hypercalcemia, renal dysfunction, and osteoporosis. *Synonym*: Burnett's syndrome.

Milroy disease: A type of familial lymphedema that causes permanent pitting in one leg initially and may affect the contralateral leg. *Synonym*: Meige disease.

Milwaukee brace: A brace used to treat adolescent idiopathic scoliosis that contains a neck ring, a trunk frame with pads to shape the curve, and a pelvic girdle. It is also called a cervicothoracolumbosacral orthosis (CTLSO) (*see* Appendix 18).

Minerva jacket: A brace or cast used to treat scoliosis that includes the head and trunk; used for cervical spine fractures or spine deformities. Also known as a Minerva cervical orthosis (*see* Appendix 18).

minimally invasive surgery (MIS): A type of surgical procedure that minimizes the size of the incision and uses specialized techniques and instrumentation.

minimal risk: The probability and magnitude that harm and discomfort anticipated in research are not greater than those ordinarily encountered in daily life or during the performance of routine physical or psychological examinations or tests.

mode: A number in a set of values that occurs most frequently. One of the measures of central tendency.

modular implant: A surgical implant where some segments are interchangeable to produce a final product that is stable.

monoarticular: Involving only one joint. Commonly used to describe types of arthritis.

monobloc implant: A type of implant that is made in one piece with no modularity.

monocyte: A circulating phagocytic leukocyte that can differentiate into a macrophage upon migrating into tissue.

mononeuropathy: Disease or damage to a single nerve; also described as a peripheral neuropathy.

monoplanar external fixation: A device that uses pins placed in bones and linear, external bars to stabilize fractures and osteotomies.

monoplegia: Paralysis only involving one limb.

monosodium urate crystals: Crystals often present in gout that are needle shaped and strongly negatively birefringent.

monostotic fibrous dysplasia: A form of fibrous dysplasia that only affects a single bone.

Monteggia fracture: A fracture pattern in the forearm where there is a break in the ulna with a dislocation of the radial head (*see* Appendix 15).

Montreal positioner: An orthopedic device used to hold patients on their side when performing procedures around the hip and pelvis by fixing pegs to a baseboard.

morbidity: Illness or abnormal condition.

Morel-Lavallée lesion: A closed traumatic soft tissue degloving where the skin and subcutaneous tissue is separated from the fascia, often found overlying the buttocks. It is associated with high-energy pelvis or acetabular fractures and is a high risk for infection.

Morquio disease: One of the mucopolysaccharidoses (type IV) that is autosomal recessive and results in the buildup of keratan sulfate. Type A is a deficiency of galactose-6-sulfate sulfatase and type B is a deficiency of beta-galactosidase. Patients may present with skeletal dysplasia, valgus knees, hypermobile joints, spinal cord compression, and cardiomegaly.

Morse taper: A method of holding 2 components together by contact friction when one implant with a shaped taper is fitted inside a matched implant. An example of a Morse taper is when a femoral stem from a hip prosthesis is fitted inside a metal head implant.

mortality: Death.

mortise view: A radiographic view that visualizes the articulating surfaces of the tibiotalar joint by internally rotating the ankle.

Morton foot: A type of foot where the first metatarsal is shorter than the second metatarsal, which may result in pain when pressure is applied to the forefoot and the head of the second metatarsal. Also referred to as a Greek foot.

Morton neuroma: A painful thickening of nerve tissue between the third and fourth metatarsal bones. Also known as Morton's toe.

motor control: The ability of the central nervous system to control or direct the neuromotor system in purposeful movement and postural adjustment by selective allocation of muscle tension across appropriate joint segments.

motor neuron: A nerve cell located on the anterior horn of the spine that sends signals from the brain to muscles.

mucopolysaccharidosis (MPS): A group of 9 hereditary and metabolic disorders in which there is a malfunction or deficiency of specific lysosomal enzymes that break down glycosaminoglycans. The syndrome types are as follows: MPS I, Hurler syndrome; MPS II, Hunter syndrome; MPS III, Sanflippo syndrome; MPS IV, Morquio disease; MPS V, Ullrich-Scheie syndrome; MPS VI, Maroteaux-Lamy syndrome; MPS VII, Sly syndrome; MPS VIII, DiFerrante syndrome; and MPS IX, Natowicz syndrome.

mucopurulent: Any discharge that appears to be mucous and infected.

multiplanar external fixation: A device that uses pins placed in bones in multiple directions and external bars to stabilize fractures and osteotomies.

multiple epiphyseal dysplasia (MED): An inherited congenital abnormality in which there is abnormal ossification at the ends of long bones, which may result in joint pain, gait abnormalities, and short limb dwarfism. The autosomal recessive form may also present with scoliosis or malformations of the hand, feet, or knees. Two types include Fairbanks disease and Ribbing disease.

multiple hereditary exostoses (MHE): An autosomal dominant disease in which patients form many benign osteochondromas, or cartilage-capped bony growths, especially around the metaphyses of long bones. May become malignant and transform to chondrosarcomas. *Synonyms*: Hereditary multiple exostosis, multiple osteochondromatosis.

multiple myeloma (MM): A malignant growth of plasma cells in the bone marrow that results in the overproduction of monoclonal paraprotein (M protein). It is the most common primary tumor found in bone where lesions appear in the spine, skull, and pelvis, which may lead to pathological fractures.

multiple regression: A statistical analysis making predictions of one variable based on measures of 2 or more other variables.

Mumford procedure: A resection of the distal clavicle to treat acromioclavicular arthritis. Can be performed open or arthroscopically.

Munster brace: A removable static brace to reduce forearm and wrist motion that is designed like a sugar tong splint, where the wrist and elbow are immobilized (*see* Appendix 18).

muscle: A bundle of fibrous tissue composed of fibrils that contract and relax to produce motion.

muscle strength: The force generated by a single maximal isometric contraction evaluated by neurologic or resistance testing, graded according to the Medical Research Council Scale (*see* Appendix 12).

muscle tone: The amount of tension or contractibility among the motor units of a muscle; often defined as the resistance of a muscle to stretch or elongate.

mutation: An error in gene replication that results in a change in the molecular structure of genetic material.

myalgia: Pain in a muscle or muscles.

myasthenia gravis: An autoimmune neuromuscular disorder in which acetylcholine receptors are blocked by antibodies at neuromuscular junctions that results in progressive muscular weakness. Patients are treated with cholinesterase inhibitors or immunosuppressants.

myelin: The white lipid that forms the principal component of the sheath of nerve cell axons in the central nervous system. Myelin increases the conduction velocity of the neuronal impulse and forms the white matter of the brain and spinal cord.

myelogram: A radiographic image of the spine after injection of a radiopaque dye; may be x-ray or computed tomography (CT). A CT myelogram may be used to assess the spinal cord and nerves if magnetic resonance imaging (MRI) is contraindicated (ie, patients with pacemakers).

myelomeningocele: A severe form of spina bifida in which the posterior elements of the spinal column do not unite (laminae) and both the meninges and spinal cord protrude posteriorly. Often associated with loss of neurologic function below the affected level. Also known as meningomyelocele and myelodysplasia.

myelopathy: Abnormality of the spinal cord due to compression (eg, central herniated disc), radiation damage, or diabetes.

myeloschisis: The most severe form of spina bifida in which the posterior elements of the spinal column do not form and there are no intact meninges, which leaves a flattened spinal cord exposed. This predisposes patients to life-threatening infections.

myoclonus: Sudden, quick spasms of a muscle group.

myoelectric prosthesis: An artificial limb with electrodes that attach to the muscles in an amputation stump, where contraction of the muscles results in limb function. This prosthesis is often used in the upper extremity.

myofibril: A fiber of muscle.

myofibrosis: Scarring in a muscle.

myolysis: Muscle breakdown.

myoma: Benign tumor consisting of muscle tissue.

myoneural junction: The junction between neurons and muscles. Also known as the neuromuscular junction.

myopathy: A disease of muscle.

myosin: A protein in muscles.

myositis: Inflammation of muscles.

myositis ossificans: Pathological growth of bone within muscle, often due to trauma, hypercalcemia, comas, and surgical intervention. *Synonym:* Heterotopic ossification.

myotonic dystrophy: An autosomal dominant trinucleotide repeat disorder that is characterized by muscle weakness and atrophy, especially of the face and neck, as well as cataracts and heart conduction defects.

myxoid chondrosarcoma: A malignant sarcoma composed of chondroblasts that contains mucus elements. Also known as a chondromyxosarcoma.

myxoma: A benign tumor composed of mucous tissue.

nail: A surgical implant that is placed within the medullary canal of a bone to fix a fracture or osteotomy. *Synonym*: Rod.

nail fold: The rounded skin surrounding each nail (for both fingernails and toenails).

nail-patella syndrome: An autosomal dominant disorder that results in underdeveloped nails and patellas. This can lead to recurrent patella dislocations, and patients may also present with webbing of the elbow and scoliosis. Also known as hereditary onychoostedysplasia, iliac horn syndrome, Turner–Kieser syndrome, or Fong disease.

naproxen: A nonsteroidal anti-inflammatory drug (NSAID), also known as naproxen sodium, that inhibits both cyclooxygenase (COX)-1 and COX-2 to reduce inflammation. Also available in different formulations in over-the-counter drugs.

Natowicz syndrome: One of the mucopolysaccharidoses (type IX) in which there is a deficiency of hyaluronidase that results in the accumulation of hyaluronic acid. Patients may present with multiple soft tissues masses, especially around joints; bony erosion; short stature; facial changes; and normal intelligence.

natural killer (NK) cell: A large granular lymphocyte capable of killing certain tumors and virally infected cells.

navicular: A bone in the foot named for its likeness to a boat. Also another name for the scaphoid, which is referred to as the navicular bone in the hand.

neck righting reflex: A reflex in infants where a change in head position results in a change in body position. The absence of this reflex often indicates developmental delay.

Chen AF, ed.
Quick Reference Dictionary for Orthopedics (pp 118-123).

neck shaft angle: The angle between the femoral neck and shaft, which is normally between 130 and 140 degrees.

necrosis: Death of tissue usually resulting in gangrene.

necrotic: Dead or avascular; normally refers to tissue.

needle: A pointed surgical device used to pass suture material through tissue. May be free (without suture) or with preattached suture.

needle biopsy: Using a needle to remove a small amount of tissue for pathologic evaluation under a microscope.

Neer classification: A fracture classification system for proximal humerus fractures based on the fracture fragments and displacement of the fragments (*see* Appendix 15).

Neer prosthesis: An orthopedic implant that is a proximal humerus replacement and is used to treat fractures or glenohumeral arthritis.

Neer sign: A clinical exam finding for subacromial impingement when a Neer test is performed after a lidocaine injection in the subacromial space and the patient's pain is decreased or absent.

Neer test: A physical exam that tests for subacromial impingement under the coracoacromial arch, which is positive when pain is elicited when the arm is in full flexion and the arm is pronated.

negative predictive value: Statistical term indicating the probability that a patient with a negative test is truly negative.

negligence: Commission of an act that a prudent person would not have done or the omission of a duty that a prudent person would have fulfilled, resulting in injury or harm to another person.

neonate: A newborn infant.

neoplasm: New and abnormal growth of tissue that may be benign or malignant; often used to describe cancer.

neoplastic fracture: A break in bone that is weakened by tumor.

nephrotoxicity: The quality of being toxic or destructive to renal cells. May be a side effect of some commonly used orthopedic drugs, including gentamicin.

nerve conduction test: Measurement of electrical conductivity of motor and sensory nerves by application of an external electrical stimulus to the nerve and evaluation of parameters such as nerve conduction time, velocity, amplitude, and shape of the resulting response as recorded from another site on the nerve or from a muscle supplied by the nerve.

nervous system: A network of nerve cells and fibers that controls and coordinates the function and movement of the body.

neuralgia: Pain along the entire course or branch of a peripheral sensory nerve.

neuralgic amyotrophy: Muscle atrophy as a result of nerve dysfunction.

neurectomy: Surgical cutting of a nerve.

neuritis: Inflammation of a nerve that leads to neuralgia.

neurofibroma: A soft tissue tumor formed in Schwann cells or neural crest cells that results in nerve enlargement.

neurofibromatosis (NF): A genetic disorder in which multiple neurofibromas are formed.

neurofibromatosis type I: The most common neurofibromatosis, in which there is a mutation in neurofibomin on chromosome 17 that results in café au lait spots, harmatomas of the iris (Lisch nodules), optic glioma, and multiple neurofibromas. *Synonym*: von Recklinghausen disease.

neurofibromatosis type II: The less common neurofibromatosis in which there is a mutation in merlin on chromosome 22 that results in bilateral acoustic neuromas (schwannoma). Also called multiple inherited schwannomas, meningiomas, and ependymomas (MISME) syndrome.

neurogenic: Something that originates from the nervous system.

neurogenic pain: Pain in the limbs caused by neurologic lesions.

neurolysis: Destruction of nerve tissue or loosening of adhesions surrounding a nerve.

neuroma: Tumor or growth along the course of a nerve or at the end of a lacerated nerve, which is often very painful.

neuromuscular junction: The junction between neurons and muscles. Also known as the myoneural junction.

neuron: Nerve cell.

neuropathy: Any disease or dysfunction of the nerves.

neuropraxia: The least severe form of damage to a nerve, in which there is a temporary loss of sensory and motor function due to nerve conduction transmission interruption.

neurorrhaphy: A surgical procedure where the nerve endings are sutured together.

neurosyphillis: A late syphilis infection in the spinal cord or brain caused by the spirochete bacteria *Treponema pallidum* that often presents 10 to 20 years after the initial infection. Patients often present with gait abnormalities, dementia, peripheral numbness, and visual disturbances (Argyll Robertson pupils). Also called tabes dorsalis.

neurotmesis: The most severe form of nerve damage, in which there is a complete transection of the nerve and the nerve sheath.

neurovascular: Involvement of both the nerves and the blood vessels.

neutrophil: A phagocytic leukocyte characterized by a multilobed nucleus and many intracellular granules.

nidus: A focal point that can be physiologically normal (eg, where a nerve begins) or abnormal (eg, where an infection begins).

Niemann-Pick disease: A severe lysosomal storage disease in which there is an accumulation of sphingomyelin that results in hepatosplenomegaly (enlargement of the liver and spleen), cherry red spots on the retina, and progressive neurological deterioration.

nightstick fracture: A fracture in the midshaft of the ulna due to direct trauma. Caused by raising the arm to block a direct overhead blow.

ninety–ninety (90–90) traction: An older method of treating femur fractures in which the hip and knee are both flexed to 90 degrees and traction is longitudinally pulled through a pin placed in the distal femur bone.

nociceptor: A peripheral nerve ending that appreciates and transmits painful or injurious stimuli.

nominal (or categorical) data: Statistical definition of data where numbers are utilized to name mutually exclusive categories.

nondisplaced fracture: A fracture in the bone that has not shifted and maintains anatomic alignment.

noninvasive test: A test that does not penetrate the skin and does not permanently change human tissue.

nonmaleficence: The medically ethical act of avoiding doing harm to another individual or creating a circumstance in which harm could occur. One part of the Hippocratic Oath.

nonossifying: A description for tumors where lesions do not create bone.

nonossifying fibroma: A benign and often asymptomatic tumor in bone that arises due to a defect in periosteal cortical bone development that leads to a failure of ossification. This fibrous cortical defect is often found in the metaphyseal and diaphyseal junction. When the lesion encompasses greater than 50% of the bone, there is a greater risk of fracture.

nonparametrics: Statistical tests that do not predict the population parameter, μ, or normality of the underlying population distribution.

nonsteroidal anti-inflammatory drug (NSAID): A pharamacologic agent that decreases inflammation by inhibiting the cyclooxygenase (COX)-1 and/or COX-2 pathway, which reduces the production of prostaglandins. An example of an NSAID is aspirin.

nonsuppurative osteomyelitis: An infection in the bone where there is no pus.

nonunion: When a fracture fails to heal or unite; may be hypertrophic, oligotrophic, or atrophic.

nonweight bearing (NWB): A restriction on activity where a patient cannot put weight on a certain extremity or extremities, often mandated to facilitate healing after sustaining a fracture or after fracture fixation.

norepinephrine: A hormone secreted by the adrenal medulla in response to splanchnic stimulation and stored in chromaffin granules. Stimulates the sympathetic nervous system and is released or administered with the patient is hypotensive.

normal distribution (or curve): A statistical description of a population that demonstrates a symmetric bell-shaped curve about the mean.

nosocomial: Disease acquired in a hospital.

noxious: Harmful to health, injurious (eg, noxious gas, noxious stimuli).

nuchal ligament: Tough, fibrous connective tissue that attaches posteriorly to the external occipital protuberance and the spinous processes of the cervical vertebrae to provide support to the neck.

nuchal rigidity: Reflex spasm of the neck extensor muscles resulting in resistance to cervical flexion.

nucleus pulposus: The inner portion of intervertebral discs composed of water and aggrecan that absorbs shocks.

null hypothesis: Statistical term indicating a hypothesis that predicts that no difference or relationship exists among the variables studied that could not have occurred by chance alone.

Ober test: A physical exam test used to determine the tightness of the iliotibial band. The patient is placed on his or her side with the affected side pointing at the ceiling and then the thigh is abducted and extended. The knee is allowed to relax, but if the flexed knee does not touch the contralateral knee, there is evidence for iliotibial (IT) band tightness.

objective measure: Method of assessment that is not influenced by the emotions or personal opinion of the assessor.

oblique fracture: A fracture pattern in which the break in the bone is slanted in relation to the long axis of the bone.

observer bias: When the opinions of an individual influence his or her observations and interpretations of behaviors being assessed or evaluated.

obstetrical palsy: A brachial plexus injury that occurs during childbirth when an infant's neck is stretched to one side during a difficult passage through the birth canal.

obturator externus: A muscle that is an external rotator of the hip. It originates from the ischiopubic rami and obturator membrane and inserts in the trochanteric fossa.

obturator internus: A muscle that is a short external rotator of the hip. It originates from the ischiopubic rami and obturator membrane and inserts in the medial greater trochanter.

obturator oblique view: One of the views of the acetabulum that is a part of the Judet views. The patient is placed supine with the involved side rotated anteriorly approximately 45 degrees with the beam aimed vertically at the involved hip. This view shows the anterior column of the acetabulum (iliopectineal line) and the posterior wall.

occlusion: Blockage or closing.

occlusive dressing: A dressing applied to a wound that prevents exposure to the air.

occult fracture: A break in the bone that is not easily identifiable by x-ray.

occupational therapy (OT): Therapeutic use of self-care, work, and play activities to increase independent function, enhance development, and prevent disability. May include adaptation of a task or environment to achieve maximum independence and to enhance the quality of life.

odontoid: The second cervical vertebrae that contains the dens, the structure around which the atlas rotates.

Ogden classification: A fracture classification system for tibial tubercle fractures (*see* Appendix 15).

olecranon: The proximal ulna that is the tip of the elbow, which articulates with the trochlea of the humerus.

oligodendroglia: Myelin-producing cells in the central nervous system.

oliguria: Diminished amount of urine formation and excretion.

olive pin: A type of pin used in Ilizarov external fixation devices where a wire with a ball on one end is used to provide compression against another fracture fragment.

Ollier disease: A condition in which multiple benign enchondromas occur in bone. Also known as enchondromatosis and dyschondroplasia.

one-tailed (directional) test: A test of the null hypothesis in which only one tail of the distribution is utilized.

onlay graft: A graft in which cortical bone is used as structural support.

open amputation: An amputation in which the distal end is not sutured closed, which permits drainage.

open biopsy: Making an incision to remove a portion of tissue for pathologic evaluation under a microscope.

open chain movements: The distal end of a kinetic chain that is not fixed.

open dislocation: A dislocation of a joint that results in interruption of the skin and exposes the joint to the air and can predispose the joint to infection.

open fracture: A break in bone where the fracture fragments disrupt the skin. Formerly referred to as a compound fracture.

open hip reduction: Relocating the femoral head inside the acetabulum by making an incision.

opening wedge osteotomy: A surgical procedure that changes bony alignment by making a partial cut in bone and placing a wedge of bone in the cut site.

open reduction: A surgical procedure in which fracture fragments are manipulated and reduced to an anatomical position through an incision.

open reduction and internal fixation (ORIF): A surgical procedure in which an incision is made and fracture bones are manipulated to an anatomical or near-anatomical position (open reduction). The fracture fragments are then held in place with hardware (internal fixation).

Oppenheim syndrome: A congenital disorder characterized by decreased muscle tone and weakness; often resolves spontaneously. *Synonyms:* Floppy baby syndrome, benign myotonia congenital.

opponensplasty: A surgical procedure in which tendons are transferred to the thumb to return function to the thumb, especially after paralysis of the opponens pollicis muscle.

opponens pollicis: A muscle that causes the thumb to oppose. It originates from the trapezium and inserts into the lateral thumb metacarpal.

opposition: The movement in which the thumb is brought across to meet the small finger.

ordinal data: Statistical description of data that is rank ordered.

origin: Proximal attachment of a muscle that remains relatively fixed during normal muscular contraction. *Antonym:* Insertion.

orthopedics: The study and treatment of musculoskeletal disorders through surgical, medical, and physical methods.

orthotic/orthosis: An external device utilized to support, position, or immobilize a part of the body, correct deformities, assist weak muscles, restore function, or modify tone. Also known as a brace.

orthotist: A person who makes and fits various braces.

Ortolani sign: A physical exam finding in congenital hip dislocation, where the hips are abducted and pressure is applied to the lateral sides of the thigh to relocate the femoral head.

os: Bone.

os acromiale: The failure of the acromion to fuse in one of the 4 ossification centers, or growth plates. May be asymptomatic or may produce pain that can limit a patient's shoulder function.

Osgood-Schlatter disease: A pathological condition in which there is inflammation of the apophysis of the tibial tubercle. Patients are often young males (11 to 15 years old) and have tenderness at the patellar tendon and proximal tibial tubercle.

osseous: Of or pertaining to bone.

ossification: The method by which bone is formed, either physiologically normal (eg, centers of ossification in bone) or abnormal (eg, heterotopic ossification in muscle).

ostectomy: The surgical removal of bone.

osteitis: Bone inflammation secondary to infection or foreign material.

osteoarthritis: A degeneration of the cartilage within a joint and the underlying bone secondary to obesity or age. Patients often present with morning stiffness and joint pain. Radiographic findings include joint space narrowing, subchondral sclerosis, and osteophytes.

osteoblast: A cell that grows into bone during development or fracture healing.

osteoblastoma: A benign tumor composed of osteoblasts in the region of calcific and osteoid tissues, often found in the spine of young patients. Also known as a giant osteoid osteoma.

osteochondral autograft transfer system (OATS) procedure: A surgical procedure that uses a patient's own cartilage from a nonweight-bearing surface to reconstitute a cartilage defect.

osteochondral defect (OCD): A lesion in the cartilage and subchondral bone secondary to excessive wear that may become displaced and result in a loose fragment within the joint. Also known as osteochondritis dissecans.

osteochondral graft: A surgical procedure to fill an osteochondral defect, where the bone and cartilage from a non-weight-bearing portion of the bone is transferred to the articular surface of the defect. The grafts are either autografts or allografts.

osteochondritis ischiopubica: Inflammation of the pubic symphysis.

osteochondroma: A benign tumor that contains bone and cartilage that is in continuity with the medullary canal; often found at the ends of long bones.

osteochondromatosis: Small cartilage formations within the synovial membrane that may be detached and enter the joint as loose bodies.

osteochondrosarcoma: A malignant tumor containing bone and cartilage.

osteochondrosis: A disease of one or more of the growth or ossification centers in children that begins as a degeneration or necrosis followed by regeneration or recalcification.

osteoclast: A large multinucleated cell that absorbs and breaks down bone.

osteoclastoma: A benign tumor of bone that contains large multinucleated cells found in the epiphysis of bones. Also known as giant cell tumor (GCT).

osteocyte: A mature osteoblast surrounded by a lacuna.

osteodystrophia deformans: A chronic disorder in which bones become thickened and deformed due to unregulated bone absorption and deposition. The 3 stages are osteoclastic activity, mixed osteoclastic and osteoblastic activity, and, finally, a burned-out stage. *Synonym*: Paget's disease.

osteodystrophy: Abnormal bone formation.

osteofibrochondrosarcoma: A malignant tumor in bone that contains osteoid, fibrous, and cartilage tissue.

osteofibroma: A benign tumor in bone that contains connective tissue.

osteogenesis imperfecta: A hereditary disorder in which there is a deficiency of type I collagen. Patients present with bones that easily fracture, blue sclerae, lax joints, and poor muscle tone. Also called brittle bones and osteitis fragilitans.

osteogenic sarcoma: Another name for osteosarcoma, which is a malignant bone tumor that demonstrates osteoblastic differentiation and malignant osteoid formation. Lesions most commonly occur in long bones (proximal tibia and humerus, distal femur).

osteoid: The unmineralized portion of bone matrix that has not undergone calcification.

osteoid osteoma: A benign bone tumor that presents with night pain and can be differentiated by a characteristic nidus seen on x-ray.

osteolysis: Bone destruction or absorption, due to disease, infection, avascular necrosis, or particle wear.

osteoma: A benign slow-growing tumor of well-differentiated bone often found on the skull or mandible.

osteomalacia: Softening of bone secondary to a lack of bone mineralization. Bones may deform or fracture with little trauma. Often caused by vitamin D deficiency, renal disease, liver disease, medications, or disorders of vitamin D metabolism. In children the term used is rickets.

osteomyelitis: A bone infection that is acute or chronic. Often treated with intravenous (IV) antibiotics.

osteon: The functional unit within cortical bone, also known as the Haversian system. In the center of the system is a Haversian canal, which is surrounded by lamellae. Osteocytes live within the lamellae and connect with each other and the Haversian canal through canaliculi.

osteonecrosis: Bone death that results from lack of blood supply to bone. Also known as avascular necrosis.

osteopenia: A disease in which there is decreased calcium in bone that produces a low bone mineral density score (T-score between −1 and −2.5). These scores are 1 to 2.5 standard deviations below an average 30-year-old White woman's bone mineral density.

osteoperiostitis: Pathologic inflammation of the periosteum, or the soft tissue covering bone.

osteopetrosis: A rare condition characterized by abnormal thickening of the bone leading to increased bone density and increased fragility of the bones. The canal may narrow significantly and bone marrow production may be compromised. Also known as Albers-Schönberg disease, marble bones, and osteosclerosis fragilis.

osteophyte: An outgrowth of bone due to cartilage degeneration within a joint or at the end of a vertebra; often seen in osteoarthritis and other inflammatory conditions. Also known as a bone spur.

osteopoikilosis: An autosomal dominant, benign sclerosing of bone, seen on x-ray as dense areas within bone.

osteoporosis: A disease in which there is significantly decreased calcium in bone that produces a very low bone mineral density score (T-score below −2.5). This score is 2.5 standard deviations below an average 30-year-old White woman's bone mineral density. Patients with osteoporosis are at increased risk for fracture and may present with stooped backs.

osteoradionecrosis: Bone death as a result of radiation, often seen in bone surrounding tumor treated with radiation therapy.

osteosarcoma: A malignant bone tumor that histologically exhibits osteoblastic differentiation and malignant osteoid formation. Lesions are most commonly seen in long bones (proximal tibia and humerus, distal femur). Also known as osteogenic sarcoma.

osteosclerosis: Thickening of the bone seen on x-ray due to increased bone density. May be due to osteoarthritis, osteopetrosis, osteopoikilosis, or hepatitis C.

osteosis: Bone formation that is abnormal.

osteosynthesis: Fracture fixation using an incision (open reduction) and holding the fracture in place with implantable devices (internal fixation).

osteotome: A surgical instrument shaped like a chisel used to cut bone. May be curved or straight and comes in a variety of widths.

osteotomy: A surgical cut of bone.

Otto disease: Protrusio, or protrusion of the femoral head through the acetabulum into the pelvis.

pachyonychia: Thickening of nails due to age or fungal infections.

Paget disease: A disorder in which bones are thickened and deformed due to unregulated bone absorption and deposition. The 3 stages of activity are osteoclastic activity, mixed osteoclastic and osteoblastic activity, and, finally, a burned-out stage. *Synonym*: Osteodystrophia deformans.

pain quality: A description of the nature, type, or character of pain that may help describe the source of pain (eg, burning: neuropathic pain; sharp: traumatic pain).

pain scale: An intensity measurement of pain that is rated on the visual analog scale where 0 is no pain and 10 is the greatest pain.

paired t test: Statistical test between 2 sample means in which selection of one sample is dependent on the other sample.

palliative care: Care rendered to temporarily reduce or moderate the intensity of an otherwise chronic medical condition.

pallor: Paleness; absence of skin coloration.

palm: The volar surface of the hand.

palmar: Location description of the palm of the hand.

palmaris brevis: A muscle that protects the ulnar nerve. It originates from the transverse carpal ligament and inserts to the medial skin of the hand.

palmaris longus: A muscle that is a weak wrist flexor that is missing in approximately 15% of the population. If present, it is commonly used as a tendon graft.

palpate: To examine by touching or feeling.

palsy: The loss of movement or ability to control movement.

Panner disease: Osteochondrosis of the capitellum of the distal humerus. Often occurs in the dominant elbow of boys between the ages of 5 and 12.

pantalar arthrodesis: A surgical fusion of the talonavicular joint (between the talus and navicular) and the subtalar joint (between the talus and calcaneus) for severe ankle and hindfoot arthritis.

paracentesis: Inserting a needle into a cavity for fluid aspiration or injection. Commonly performed in the abdomen.

paraffin bath: A modality of heat therapy where hands or feet are bathed in warm paraffin to facilitate increased range of motion.

paralysis: Condition in which one loses voluntary motor control over a section of the body due to trauma or injury.

paraplegia: Condition in which the lower half of the body (trunk and lower extremities) is paralyzed due to spinal cord injury below the cervical spine.

parasympathetic nervous system: Autonomic nervous system that serves to relax the body's responses and is the opposite of the sympathetic nervous system.

paraxial: Lying near the axis of the body.

paraxial hemimelia: Congenital absence of all or part of one of the bones in the forearm (radius or ulna) or leg (tibia or fibula).

paravertebral muscle spasm: An involuntary muscle contraction of the muscles surrounding the lower spine.

parenchyma: Essential parts of an organ containing specialized cell types (eg, hepatocytes in liver).

parenteral: Administration by subcutaneous, intramuscular, or intravenous injection, thereby bypassing the gastrointestinal tract.

paresis: Weakness in voluntary muscle with slight paralysis.

paresthesia: Abnormal sensation, such as burning, pricking, tickling, or tingling. Commonly seen in extremities of diabetic patients.

Parkinson disease: A degenerative neurological condition in which cells in the substantia nigra die, which reduces the amount of dopamine produced. Patients often present with cogwheel rigidity, tremors, shuffling gait, and dementia.

paronychia: An inflammation of the tissues surrounding a nail.

parosteal sarcoma: Malignant tumor of the periosteum, most commonly occurring on the surface of the metaphysis of long bone. Often found in the posterior distal femur and the proximal humerus.

pars interarticularis: The portion of the spinal vertebrae that connects the superior and inferior articular facets; also known as pars.

partial articular-sided tendon avulsion (PASTA) lesion: A lesion of the shoulder where the intra-articular portion of the rotator cuff is partially torn.

partial thromboplastin time (PTT): A measurement of clotting that determines the time it takes for a blood sample to clot when the intrinsic clotting cascade is chemically activated. Heparin is an example of a drug that prolongs the PTT.

partial weight bearing (PWB): A restriction in activity where a patient can only place a portion of his or her weight through a specified extremity, often denoted by a percentage.

passive range of motion (PROM): Amount of motion at a given joint when the joint is moved by an individual besides the patient.

passive stretch: Stretch applied with an external force. May be a sign of compartment syndrome with pain with passive stretch applied by the clinician.

patella: The bone in the anterior portion of the knee that contributes to the extensor mechanism of the leg. It is the largest sesmoid bone in the body and is commonly called the kneecap.

patellectomy: Removal of a portion or the entire patella.

patellofemoral arthroplasty: A replacement of the patellofemoral joint with a prosthesis due to isolated arthritis between the patella and the femur.

patellofemoral disease: A common cause of anterior knee pain where the patella articulates with the femur. It may be due to patellar malalignment, chondromalacia of the patella, or subluxation of the patella. Treatment often consists of quadriceps strengthening, specifically vastus medialis oblique (VMO) exercises.

pathogen: Any disease-producing agent or microorganism.

pathognomonic: Something that is characteristic for a particular disease.

pathologic fracture: A break in a bone that is weakened by infection, tumor, surgery, or injury.

pathology: The study of the characteristics, causes, and effects of disease, as observed in the structure and function of the body.

Pauwel classification: A fracture classification system for femoral neck fractures based on the angle of the fracture (*see* Appendix 15).

Pavlik harness: A brace used to treat congenital hip dislocations in an infant, where both legs are placed in the harness, the hips and knees are flexed, and the legs are abducted. May also be used to treat femur fracture in infants (*see* Appendix 18).

Pearson r: Statistical technique that shows the degree of relationship between variables (also called the product-moment correlation).

pectineus: A muscle that flexes and adducts the hip. It originates from the pectineal line of the pubis to the pectineal line of the femur.

pectus carinatum: Undue prominence of the sternum; also called chicken or pigeon chest or breast.

pectus excavatum: Undue depression of the sternum; also called funnel chest or breast.

pedicle: (1) A portion of tissue attached by a stalk, which provides the tissue support or nutrients. (2) The portion of the spine vertebra that connects the anterior and posterior elements of the vertebra. Often the location of screw fixation in the spine.

pedicle flap: A type of flap where tissue is transplanted from another location with the blood vessels still attached to it.

peer review: Appraisal by professional coworkers of equal status regarding how health practitioners conduct practice, education, or research.

pegboard: A type of surgical positioning device that can hold a patient in a lateral decubitus position using a board with holes. Often used in total hip arthroplasty cases.

Pellegrini-Stieda disease: Calcification noted on the medial collateral ligament (MCL) of the knee, often noted on x-ray and due to trauma or chronic irritation.

pelvic binder: A brace applied over the greater trochanters of both femurs to provide compression and to initially stabilize a pelvic ring fracture in a hemodynamically unstable patient if there is suspected bleeding.

pelvic girdle: The bony arch that provides support to the legs, including the pelvis and femur.

pelvic inlet view: A caudal projection of the pelvis where one can best see the pelvic ring to evaluate for findings, such as opening of the pubic symphysis and posterior displacement of the ring.

pelvic outlet view: A cephalad projection of the pelvis where one can best see the hemipelvis to assess for vertical shift of the pelvis.

Pemberton osteotomy: A surgical procedure performed to treat congenital hip dislocation by incompletely cutting the transiliac bone and rotating the bone to better cover the femoral head in the acetabulum.

percutaneous pinning: Insertion of hardware to fix a fracture without having to make a skin incision.

perfusion: The act of pouring over or through, especially the passage of a fluid through the vessels of a specific organ or body part.

periarticular: The area surrounding a joint.

perilunate dislocation: Dislocation of the lunate in the wrist, which requires closed or open reduction.

periosteum: The soft tissue encasing long bone that provides a vascular supply to the bone. In children, the periosteum is stronger and thicker and may contribute to bone growth.

peripheral nervous system (PNS): Consists of all of the nerve cells outside the central nervous system, including motor and sensory nerves.

peripheral neuropathy: Any functional or organic disorder of the peripheral nervous system; degeneration of peripheral nerves supplying the extremities, causing loss of sensation, muscle weakness, and atrophy.

peripheral vascular system: The blood vessels that supply the arms and legs.

peroneal: Related to the fibula.

peroneus: The fibula, or the smaller of the 2 bones in the leg.

peroneus brevis: A muscle in the lateral compartment of the leg that everts the foot. It originates from the distal lateral fibula and inserts in the base of the fifth metatarsal.

peroneus longus: A muscle in the lateral compartment of the leg that everts and plantarflexes the foot. It originates from the proximal lateral fibula and inserts in the plantar surface of the base of the first metatarsal.

peroneus tertius: A muscle in the anterior compartment of the leg that dorsiflexes and everts the foot. It originates from the distal fibula and interosseous membrane and inserts in the base of the fifth metatarsal.

Perthes disease: Another name for Legg-Calvé-Perthes (LCP) disease, where the capital femoral epiphysis undergoes spontaneous avascular necrosis in children that leads to flattening and collapse of the femoral head.

pes: The foot.

pes anserinus: The confluence of the sartorius, gracilus, and semitendinosus muscles onto the anteromedial portion of the tibia. Stands for "goose foot" in French. May develop a bursitis over the area. Often used as the site of hamstring graft harvesting.

phalangectomy: The surgical removal of one of the phalanxes in the finger or toes.

phalanges: Bones of the fingers and toes.

phantom limb pain: Paresthesia or severe pain felt in the amputated part of a limb.

pharmacokinetics: The study of how the body handles drugs, including the way in which drugs are absorbed, distributed, and eliminated.

phlebitis: Inflammation of a vein.

phlebothrombosis: Clotting or thrombosis within a vein.

phocomelia: A defect in the development of an extremity in which the hands or feet are either attached directly to the trunk or with poorly developed bone. Often due to genetics or the use of thalidomide, a drug that was previously used to treat morning sickness.

phrenic nerve: The nerve that innervates the diaphragm and contains branches from cervical roots 3, 4, and 5 (memory hint: C3, 4, and 5 keep the diaphragm alive).

physeal fracture: Fracture pattern through a growth plate. *Synonym*: Salter-Harris fracture.

physical therapy (PT): Treatment of injury and disease by mechanical means, such as heat, light, exercise, massage, and mobilization.

physician assistant (PA): Health professional licensed or, in the case of those employed by the federal government, credentialed to practice medicine with physician supervision.

physis: The location of bone growth. The 4 zones in a physis are as follows: resting cartilage zone, proliferating cartilage zone, the zone of hypertrophy, and the zone of calcification.

piezoelectric effect: The ability of certain materials to convert mechanical energy from compression into electrical energy.

pigeon-toed: A physical exam finding where the feet are internally rotated due to tibial torsion.

pigmented villonodular synovitis (PVNS): A benign condition in which the synovial lining of a joint, most commonly the knee and hip, becomes hyperplastic, which results in large effusions and bony erosions.

pilon fracture: A fracture pattern of the articulating surface of the distal tibia (within 5 cm of the joint line) that is often the result of an impaction force and axial load to the leg. May be associated with a fibula fracture.

pin: A threaded and enlongated surgical implant often made of stainless steel that is used to stabilize bone (for an external fixator), to pull traction (distal femur or proximal tibia traction pin), and to aid in fracture fixation.

pincer deformity: A form of femoroacetabular impingement in which there is excess bone formation on the acetabulum that results in abnormal contact with the femoral head.

pinch test: A test of finger strength measured by squeezing a fingertip to the thumb. Decreased pinch test strength is due to ulnar nerve dysfunction.

pin tract infection: A type of infection that occurs around the pins used in external fixation devices, especially because contaminants may travel from the outside of the pin down to bone and soft tissue.

Pipkin classification: A classification for fractures of the femoral head and the association with hip dislocations (*see* Appendix 15).

piriformis: A muscle that is an external rotator of the hip.

piriformis syndrome: A condition characterized by overactivity of the piriformis muscle (one of the short external rotators of the hip), causing external rotation of the leg and buttock pain.

piroxicam: A type of nonsteroidal anti-inflammatory drug (NSAID) that is a nonselective cyclooxygenase (COX) inhibitor. It is available in oral, intravenous, and ointment forms.

pistol grip deformity: A radiographic sign of femoroacetabular impingement, where the proximal femur has an abnormal shape that is described to look like the grip of a pistol.

pivot shift test: A physical exam test for the stability of the anterior cruciate ligament (ACL). The patient is placed supine on the examination table, the hip is flexed to 30 degrees, and the tibia is internally rotated 20 degrees. A valgus force is applied to the knee while it is flexed. The ACL may be incompetent if the tibia subluxes on the femur.

plafond: The distal part of the tibia that articulates with the talus. Derived from French: flat (plat) bottom (fond).

plantar: The bottom portion of the foot.

plantar fasciitis: Inflammation of the plantar fascia, or the aponeurosis on the sole of the foot that forms a part of the arch.

plantar fibromatosis: Plantar fascia scarring that produces painful nodules along the plantar surface of the feet. *Synonym:* Lederhosen disease.

plantarflexion: Moving the foot at the ankle downward and away from the body.

plantaris: A muscle with a small muscle belly and long tendon that originates from the lateral femoral condyle and attaches to the calcaneus that assists with plantarflexing the foot. The tendon passes the lateral and posterior border of the knee.

planus: Flat.

plasma cell: Mature antibody-secreting cell derived from the B cell. Overproduction of plasma cells is the cause of multiple myeloma.

plate: An orthopedic implant used for fracture fixation that is a sheet of metal with holes for screw fixation that can be malleable or rigid.

plateau fracture: An intra-articular fracture of the flat portion of the bone, often referring to a fracture of the proximal tibia. May be diagnosed by imaging or aspirating synovial fluid. If there is trauma but no fracture, the synovial fluid will be bloody; if there is a plateau fracture, the synovial fluid will be bloody and have fat due to extravasated bone marrow.

platelets: Cells within the circulatory system that lead to the formation of blood clots. They are derived from megakaryocytes and do not have nuclei. Also known as thrombocytes.

platform crutches: Crutches designed to redirect stress during ambulation from the joints in the wrist and hand to the forearm. May be used to aid some individuals with ambulation who are non-weight bearing in one upper and one lower extremity.

platysma: The superficial neck muscle that is innervated by cranial nerve VII (facial nerve) and controls depression of the mouth. This area is dissected when doing an anterior cervical discectomy and fusion (ACDF).

pleomorphic undifferentiated sarcoma (PUS): The current name for malignant fibrous histiocytoma (MFH), a soft tissue sarcoma with undifferentiated cells and no cell or origin. *Synonym*: Undifferentiated pleomorphic sarcoma.

plexus: An intricate network of vessels or nerves.

plica: A folded segment of synovium within a joint.

plica syndrome: Irritation to and inflammation of a plica, most commonly seen in the medial patellofemoral plica in the knee. May be treated conservatively or through arthroscopic plica resection.

pneumoarthrogram: An injection of air into a joint seen on x-ray fluoroscopy that outlines the articular surface of a joint. May be used in a hip arthrogram prior to injecting dye to ensure proper needle placement within the hip joint.

podiatrist: A medical specialist that specifically focuses on foot and ankle conditions.

pointer: A contusion in the front of the hip, often seen in football players. *Synonym*: Stinger.

Poland syndrome: A rare congenital abnormality in which a patient is born without a pectoralis major muscle and has syndactyly of the ipsalateral hand.

poliomyelitis: Viral infection of the motor cells in the spinal cord. Also known as polio.

pollicization: A surgical procedure in which a finger (often the index finger) is made into an opposable thumb. Often performed in patients born without a functional thumb or in patients with traumatic thumb amputations who are not able to undergo other thumb reconstruction options (eg, toe to thumb transfers).

polyarthritis: Arthritis in 2 or more joints.

polydactyly: A congenital anomaly in which there are more than 5 fingers or toes on each extremity.

polyethylene (PE): The plastic used in orthopedic implants, such as acetabular liners and knee replacements. Various manufacturing processing options exist, including cross-linking and molding versus ram-extruding the implants. Sterilization is currently conducted using gamma irradiation in an oxygen-free environment but has historically been done with gas plasma, ethylene oxide, and gamma irradiation in air. Currently, antioxidants, such as vitamin E, have been added to PE to reduce free radicals that can cause osteolysis.

polymethylmethacrylate (PMMA): A viscoelastic cement used in orthopedics that is biologically compatible and acts as a space-filling and load-transferring material that mechanically bonds to cancellous bone. It is used for implant fixation, antibiotic spacers, and to fill voids. PMMA can heat to greater than 80°C when hardening, which can cause thermal necrosis.

polymyositis: Systemic connective tissue disease characterized by inflammatory and degenerative changes in the muscles. It leads to symmetric weakness and some degree of muscle atrophy; its etiology is unknown.

polyneuritis: Inflammation of many nerves at once.

polyneuropathy: A disease involving several nerves such as that seen in diabetes mellitus.

polyostotic fibrous dysplasia: A hereditary disease characterized by fibrous dysplasia lesions, precocious puberty in females, and multiple café au lait spots. *Synonyms:* McCune-Albright syndrome.

polypharmacy: The excessive and unnecessary use of medications.

polypropylene: The plastic used to make braces and orthotics.

Ponseti casting: A method of treating clubfoot through serial castings. The order of correction is as follows: (1) cavus, (2) adduction, (3) heel varus, and (4) equinus.

popliteal cyst: A sac of synovial fluid in the back of the knee (popliteal fossa) that is often seen in osteoarthritic knees. *Synonym:* Baker cyst.

popliteal fossa: The area behind the knee shaped like a diamond and bordered by the 2 heads of the gastrocnemius, as well as the semimembranosus, semitendinosus, and biceps femoris. The contents include the popliteal artery and vein, the common peroneal nerve, the tibial nerve, and popliteal lymph nodes.

popliteal nerve block: A regional delivery of local anesthetic agent from the popliteal fossa that reduces pain and sensation in the distal leg below knee (sciatic nerve distribution), except for the medial leg that is innervated by the saphenous nerve.

popliteus muscle: A muscle of the deep compartment of the leg that laterally rotates the femur in relation to the tibia during closed chain movements. It originates from the lateral femur condyle and inserts on the posterior shaft of the tibia.

popliteus tendon: The tendon of the popliteus muscle at the origin that contributes to the posterolateral corner of the knee. Visualized in the lateral compartment during arthroscopy or arthrotomy of the knee.

population: The entire sample of patients (N).

positive predictive value: Statistical term indicating the probability that a patient with a positive test is truly positive.

positron emission tomography (PET): A type of nuclear imaging that uses positron-emitting radionuclide ligands to detect functional physiology through imaging. A common ligand is fluorodeoxyglucose (FDG), which is used to identify sections of the body that have increased metabolic activity. Often used to identify tumor locations and may be used in conjunction with a computed tomography (CT) scan to provide 3D anatomic overlay with functional PET images (*see* Appendix 22).

posterior: Toward the back of the body. *Synonym*: Dorsal.

posterior cruciate ligament (PCL): Ligament that connects the femur to the tibia and prevents posterior translation and rotation of the tibia relative to the femur. May be treated nonoperatively.

posterior longitudinal ligament (PLL): A strong connective tissue band that connects vertebral bodies in the back. May be ossified (OPLL).

posteroanterior (PA): A radiographic projection where the x-ray beam passes from the back (posterior) to the front (anterior).

posterolateral corner (PLC): The posterior and lateral corner of the knee that is composed of the lateral collateral ligament (LCL), popliteus, and the popliteo-fibular ligament.

posttraumatic arthritis: A type of arthritis that results from previous injury to the cartilage (trauma, infection, etc) that predisposes the joint to further cartilage degradation. May occur after both nonoperative and operative treatment.

Pott disease: Extrapulmonary tuberculosis found in the spine, which can result in vertebral collapse and kyphosis. Most often found in the lower thoracic and upper lumbar vertebrae. Also called tuberculous spondylitis.

power: A statistical term that indicates the probability that a test will reject the null hypothesis when the null hypothesis is actually false and obtain a statistically significant effect. It is the probability that the test will not make a type II error $(1 − β)$.

Prader-Willi syndrome: A congenital disease in which some genes on the paternal chromosome 15 are not expressed, which results in morbid obesity, mental retardation, and decreased height. Orthopedic manifestations of Prader-Willi include valgus knees, developmental dysplasia of the hip, and scoliosis.

precision: Statistical term that indicates the reliability and reproducibility of an experiment.

predictive validity: Positive correlation between test scores and future performance.

prednisone: A synthetic corticosteroid that is an immunosuppressant. It may be used to treat inflammatory diseases, cancer, and conditions with low glucocorticoid levels.

preferred provider organization (PPO): Acts as a broker between the purchaser of health care and the provider.

prepatellar bursitis: Inflammation of the bursa anterior to the patella, often due to chronic or direct trauma. *Synonym*: Housemaid knee.

press-fit: A technique used in arthroplasty where implants are placed into the joint without cement to allow bone to grow into the porous rough surface of the implant.

pressure relief ankle–foot orthosis (PRAFO): A static brace that keeps the foot in 90 degrees of dorsiflexion and provides padding to the heel to prevent pressure sores (*see* Appendix 18).

pressure sore: An area of localized tissue damage caused by ischemia due to pressure.

prevalence: The total number of persons with a disease in a given population at a given point in time. Prevalence is usual expressed as the percentage of a population that has the disease.

Prieser disease: Avascular necrosis of the scaphoid, thought to be due to repetitive microtrauma or the side effects of medication.

primitive reflex (reaction): Any reflex normal in an infant or fetus. Its presence in an adult usually indicates serious neurologic disease (eg, grasp, Moro, and sucking reflexes).

process: An anatomical term used to describe a prominent part of a bone (eg, coronoid process).

prognosis: Prediction of the probable outcome given the patient's condition.

progressive resistance exercise (PRE): A method that therapists use to gradually increase the ability of muscles to generate force through exercise.

pronation: (1) Rotation of the forearm inward (medially) so that the palm is facing toward the floor. (2) For the foot, turning the plantar surface of the foot outward. Involves a combination of eversion and abduction to lower the longitudinal arch of the foot.

pronator quadratus: A muscle that pronates the forearm. It originates from the medial distal ulna and inserts in the anterior distal radius.

pronator teres: A muscle that pronates and flexes the forearm. It originates from the medial epicondyle of the humerus and coronoid process and inserts in the lateral radius.

prone: Lying face down.

prophylactic: Preventative.

proprioception: Self-awareness of posture, movement, and changes in equilibrium and the knowledge of position, weight, and resistance of objects in relation to the body.

prosthesis: Artificial substitutes, often mechanical or electrical, used to replace missing body parts.

prothrombin time (PT): A measurement of clotting through the extrinsic clotting cascade that determines the time it takes for plasma to clot after adding tissue factor. Warfarin is an example of a drug that prolongs the PT.

protrusio acetabula: Protrusion of the femur through the acetabulum. Radiographically indicated by disruption of Kohler's line. Also known as Otto disease.

proximal: Anatomic position located near to the trunk (eg, the elbow is more proximal than the wrist).

proximal femoral replacement (PFR): A replacement of the proximal femur with a megaprosthesis due to tumor, total hip arthroplasty revisions, or fracture.

proximal interphalangeal joint (PIP): The joint between the proximal and middle phalanges of a finger or toe.

proximal row carpectomy (PRC): Excision of the proximal row of the carpal bones (scaphoid, lunate, triquetrum) used to treat localized arthritis (eg, scapholunate advanced collapse [SLAC] wrist) or carpal instability.

pseudarthrosis: Nonunion at a fracture or osteotomy site, where a "false joint" is created and movement can occur around the nonhealing ends of a fracture or osteotomy site.

pseudogout: A crystal arthropathy in which calcium pyrophosphate dehydrate is deposited into joints, which are rhomboid and weakly positive birefringent when inspected under a microscope. *Synonym*: Calcium pyrophosphate dehydrate (CPPD) disease.

pseudohypoparathyroidism: A genetic condition characterized by the body's lack of response to parathyroid hormone, which results in low serum calcium and high phosphate and parathyroid hormone. In the orthopedic population, patients present with shortened fourth and fifth metacarpals. Also known as Albright's hereditary osteodystrophy and Seabright bantam syndrome.

pseudomonas: A gram-negative bacteria that is aerobic and rod shaped. The most common form found in orthopedics is *Pseudomonas aeruginosa* and it is often found in diabetic patients.

psoas muscle: A muscle that flexes the hip. It originates from the lumbar spine (L1 to L5 vertebrae) and inserts into the lesser trochanter.

psoriatic arthritis: A type of inflammatory arthritis that is associated with psoriasis.

pubic symphysis: The cartilaginous joint that connects the left and right superior rami. May undergo diastasis due to trauma or childbirth.

pulmonary embolism: An obstruction of the pulmonary artery or one of its branches usually caused by an embolus from a deep vein thrombosis. The gold standard of diagnosis is a pulmonary angiography. However, because these are very invasive, most pulmonary emboli are diagnosed with a chest computed tomography (CT) scan with contrast. Patients often present in the postoperative phase with tachypnea, tachycardia, and hypoxia. Treatment consists of pharmacologic anticoagulation and/or insertion of an inferior vena cava (IVC) filter to prevent further clots from developing in the lungs.

punctate: Having small spots, punctures, or points.

purulent: Consisting of or containing pus.

pus: Thick fluid indicative of infection containing leukocytes, bacteria, and cellular debris.

Pyle disease: An autosomal recessive disease with abnormality of bone remodeling in the metaphysis that results in expansion of the metaphysis. This most commonly occurs at the distal femur, proximal tibia, and proximal fibula. Patients may also present with scoliosis, valgus knees, and bone fragility. *Synonym*: Metaphyseal dysplasia.

pyramidal tract: Nerve tracts in the anterior portion of the spinal cord that control movement. Also known as the corticospinal tract.

pyrexia: A fever.

q angle: A measurement to determine patella subluxation or patella maltracking, where a line is drawn from the anterior superior iliac spine to the middle of the patella and then from the center of the patella to the tibia tubercle. The angle formed is the Q angle, which is normally 14 degrees in males and 17 degrees in females. A higher angle indicates a valgus angle.

quadrangular space: An axillary space in the arm that contains the axillary nerve and posterior circumflex humeral artery. The borders of the space include the subscapularis (superior), teres major (inferior), long head of the triceps brachii (medial), and humeral surgical neck (lateral).

quadratus femoris: A muscle that is a short external rotator of the hip that contains the medial femoral circumflex artery that supplies blood to the femoral head. It originates from the ischial tuberosity and inserts in the intertrochanteric crest of the femur.

quadratus plantae: A muscle that assists with toe flexion. It originates from the medial and lateral plantar calcaneus and inserts in the lateral flexor digitorum longus (FDL) tendon.

quadriceps: A complex of muscles that extends the knee composed of 4 muscles, including the rectus femoris, vastus lateralis, vastus intermedius, and vastus medialis.

quadrilateral plate: The part of bone in the adult pelvis that is composed of the ilium, ischium, and pubis, which forms the medial wall of the acetabulum.

quadriplegia: Paralysis of all 4 extremities.

qualitative research: A form of research that investigates the unique properties of a natural setting without reliance on quantitative data.

Chen AF, ed.
Quick Reference Dictionary for Orthopedics (pp 148-149).
© 2012 Taylor & Francis Group.

quality-adjusted life years (QALY): A research measurement for disease burden that accounts for the quality and quantity of life. It is used to determine the number of years of life that an intervention would add.

quality assurance (QA) project: A project conducted to ensure that quality is being maintained by constantly measuring outcomes and comparing them to a set of standards.

quality of life: The degree of satisfaction that an individual has regarding particular style of life.

quantitative: Measureable.

R

rachischisis: A congenital defect in which the neural tube does not fully close and the vertebrae are not fully formed. The spine is exposed, which leads to problems with bladder function, chronic infections, and motor and sensory deficits.

rachitis: Inflammation of the spinal column due to vitamin D deficiency.

radial deviation: Bending the hand or the wrist toward the radius.

radicular: Pertaining to a nerve root. May describe the path of pain.

radiculopathy: Damage to a nerve root that often results in pain that radiates down a dermatome distribution. May be caused by compression from a lateral or far lateral herniated disc, as well as a tumor, decreased blood supply, or inflammation. Also known as radiculitis.

radiograph: Commonly referred to as an x-ray.

radiolucent: Anything that is transparent to x-rays, such as soft tissue.

radiopaque: Anything that is not transparent to x-rays, such as metal.

radioulnar synostosis: The formation of heterotopic bone between the radius and ulna that occurs secondary to trauma, surgery, or congenital anomalies.

radius: The larger of the 2 bones of the forearm.

ramus: A branch. In anatomy, a general term to designate a smaller structure given off by a larger one (eg, ventral or dorsal rami off of spinal nerves, pubic ramus off of the pubis bone).

randomization: Process of assigning participants or objects to a control or experimental group on a random basis in order to reduce bias in a research study.

Chen AF, ed.
Quick Reference Dictionary
for Orthopedics (pp 150-155).
© 2013 Taylor & Francis Group

randomized controlled trial (RCT): A study design in which people are allocated at random (by chance) to receive one of several clinical interventions. After randomization, the 2 (or more) groups of subjects are followed in exactly the same way. RCTs are considered by most to be the most reliable form of scientific evidence in the hierarchy of evidence (levels I and II evidence).

range of motion (ROM): The path of motion a joint can move in any one direction, measured in degrees.

Ray amputation: Surgical removal of a metacarpal and associated finger or a metatarsal and associated toe.

Raynaud phenomenon: A condition of decreased blood supply to the extremities characterized by vasospasm in the fingers, toes, nose, and ears due to cold weather or various stimuli.

reactive hyperemia: Extra blood in vessels in response to a period of blocked blood flow.

reamer: A surgical cutting instrument used to widen holes in bone.

reamer irrigator aspirator (RIA): A method of obtaining bone autograft from bones with long intramedullary canals by reaming and irrigating within the canal and then aspirating bone graft and marrow and filtering it prior to reinserting it into the patient.

receptor: Specific site at which a drug acts through forming a chemical bond.

receptor activator of nuclear factor κβ (RANK): A receptor on the surface of osteoclasts that activates bone resorption when attached to RANK-L. It plays a role in bone homeostasis.

receptor activator of nuclear factor κβ ligand (RANK-L): A molecule found on the surface of osteoblasts that attaches to RANK on osteoclasts to activate bone resorption. When there is decreased RANK-L, the amount of bone resorption decreases. It plays a role in bone homeostasis.

rectus femoris: A muscle that flexes the hip and extends the knee. It is part of the quadriceps muscle that originates from the anterior inferior iliac spine and inserts on the tibial tubercle.

recurvatum: Hyperextension of the knee joint, often seen in connective tissue disease such as Marfan syndrome and Ehlers-Danlos syndrome.

red blood cell (RBC): The oxygen-carrying cell in blood that is produced in bone marrow. Packed red blood cells (PRBC) are the product of transfusion after blood loss. Also known as erythrocytes.

reduction: Realignment of a dislocated bone to its original position.

referred pain: Visceral pain felt in a somatic area away from the actual source of pain.

reflex: Involuntary reaction to an external stimulus.

reflex arc (spinal reflex arc): A reflex that travels through the spine and not to the brain. A stimulus occurs that is detected by a receptor, transmitted to a sensory neuron, passed through a relay neuron or interneuron in the spinal cord, and delivered to a motor neuron to the appropriate effector where the reflex occurs.

Regan and Morrey classification: A fracture classification system based on the amount of coronoid process fractured (*see* Appendix 15).

regression analysis: Statistical method that analyzes several variables at once, examining the relationship between independent variables and a dependent variable. This analysis determines whether a dependent variable changes when all but one of the independent variables are held constant.

rehabilitation: Helping individuals regain skills and abilities that have been lost as a result of illness, injury or disease, disorder, or incarceration.

reimplantation: A surgical procedure in which a portion of the body is reattached to the original site (eg, reimplantation of a digit after amputation).

Reiter syndrome: An autoimmune condition that is triggered by infection and presents with iridocyclitis (inflammation of the iris or the front of the eye), urethritis (inflammation of the urethra), and arthritis (rheumatoid factor [RF] negative and HLA-B27 positive). Also known as reactive arthritis (memory hint: can't see, can't pee, can't climb a tree).

reliability: Predictability of an outcome regardless of the observer.

remission: A period of time during which the symptoms of a disease are not detectable; may be permanent. Often used to describe cancer after treatment is administered.

renal osteodystrophy: A disease in which chronic kidney dysfunction leads to electrolyte abnormalities (decreased calcium, increased phosphate), which results in bone demineralization. Also known as renal rickets.

research: Systematic investigation, including development, testing, and evaluation design.

resect: To surgically remove, as in removal of tumors, tissues, or body parts.

resorption: The process of absorbing a tissue (eg, resorption of bone).

restraints: Devices used to aid in immobilizing patients, especially when they are combative.

retinaculum: A band of connective tissue that holds tissues or organs in place.

retrolisthesis: The posterior subluxation of a vertebra in relation to the vertebrae inferior to it. Often occurs in degenerative arthritis in older patients.

retroversion: An anatomic position term that describes a structure that is rotated behind or toward the back of the body. Often used to describe the femur, humerus, or acetabulum. *Antonym*: Anteversion.

reverse Trendelenburg: A position where a supine patient's bed is tilted 45 degrees so that the patient's head is above the level of his or her feet.

revision: A reoperation on a previously performed procedure.

rhabdomyoma: Benign tumor of striated muscle, often found in the heart.

rhabdomyosarcoma: Malignant tumor of striated muscle that arises from skeletal muscle.

rheumatoid arthritis (RA): An autoimmune arthritis where autoantibodies destroy connective tissue and joints, especially the knees, spine, hands, and feet.

rheumatoid factor (RF): A laboratory test that determines the amount of autoantibody against a portion of the antibody immunoglobulin G (IgG). May be elevated in infection but will have high values in patients with rheumatoid arthritis or Sjögren syndrome.

Rh factor: Hereditary blood factor found in red blood cells determined by specialized blood tests; when present, a person is Rh positive; when absent, a person is Rh negative.

rib: One of 12 pairs of bones attached to vertebrae posteriorly that curve toward the sternum and protect the thoracic cavity.

rib vertebral angle (RVA): A measurement off of x-ray to determine whether an infantile idiopathic scoliosis curve will progress. The angle is measured between the apical vertebra of the curve and either rib on the side of that vertebra. If the rib vertebral angle is greater than 20 degrees, the curve is more likely to progress. *Synonym:* Mehta angle.

RICE: An acronym to apply when treating muscle and ligament sprains: rest, ice, compress (with an elastic band), and elevate.

rickets: A spectrum of diseases caused by deficiency of or resistance to vitamin D that results in softened bone. This term is only used to describe vitamin D deficiency in children and may present as various diseases: vitamin D–resistant rickets, vitamin D–dependent rickets, congenital rickets, and nutritional rickets.

rigidity: Hypertonicity of muscles. Muscles that are unable to relax and are in a constant state of contraction, even at rest.

Riseborough and Radin classification: A fracture classification for intercondylar humerus fractures based on displacement and rotation (*see* Appendix 15).

risk factors: Factors that cause a person or group of people to be particularly vulnerable to an unhealthy event.

Risser stages: A radiographic determination of bone maturity based on the ossification of the iliac crest apophysis. There are 4 stages that describe the least to most mature bone: (1) ossification of the lateral one quarter of the crest, (2) ossification of one half of the crest, (3) ossification of three quarters of the crest, and (4) complete ossification without fusion.

rocker bottom foot: A congenital anomaly of the foot in which the talus is plantarflexed and the forefoot is dorsiflexed. It is associated with some congenital disorders, including trisomy 13 (Patau's syndrome), trisomy 18 (Edwards' syndrome), and trisomy 9. Also known as congenital vertical talus.

rod: A surgical implant placed with the medullary canal of bone for fracture or osteotomy fixation. *Synonym:* Nail.

roentgenogram: An x-ray.

Romberg sign: The inability to maintain body balance when the eyes open and then close with the feet together, which indicates a loss of proprioceptive control.

rongeur: A surgical instrument that is used to take small pieces from bone. When used in spinal surgery, it may also be referred to as a Lexel rongeur.

rotation: Movement around the long axis of a limb.

rotational flap: A flap where a section of tissue is transferred to an adjacent section carrying its own blood and nerve supply.

rotator cuff (RC): The muscle complex of the shoulder that provides stability to the glenohumeral joint and assists with shoulder abduction. The muscles that comprise the rotator cuff include the supraspinatus, infraspinatus, teres minor, and subscapularis muscle, which travel in a counterclockwise position when looking at the glenoid in a sagittal plane.

rotator cuff arthropathy: Glenohumeral arthritis that presents with a concomitant large rotator cuff tear.

rudimentary: An undeveloped part of the body.

Rüedi and Allgöwer classification: A fracture classification system for pilon fractures (*see* Appendix 15).

rupture: A bursting or the state of being broken apart.

sacral agenesis: Congenital partial or complete absence of the sacrum. Also known as caudal regression syndrome.

sacralization: The lack of fusion of S1 (sacral vertebra 1) to the sacrum, which results in an additional lumbar segment (L6). Also called lumbarization.

sacrectomy: Surgical removal of the sacrum.

sacrocoxalgia: Pain present in the sacrum and coccyx (tailbone) region.

sacrodynia: Pain in the sacrum.

sacroiliac joint: The joint between the sacrum and iliac wing that may become inflamed.

sagittal plane: A plane that runs from anterior to posterior.

salsalate: A type of nonsteroidal anti-inflammatory drug (NSAID) that may produce fewer gastrointestinal side effects.

Salter-Harris classification: A fracture classification system for physeal fractures or fractures through the growth plate. *Synonym*: Physeal fracture (*see* Appendix 15).

Salter osteotomy: A type of open wedge innominate osteotomy to treat congenital hip dislocation. The osteotomy extends and retroverts the acetabulum around a fixed axis.

sample: A portion of the population chosen for an experiment that is assumed to represent the population (n).

Sanders classification: A fracture classification system for calcaneus fractures (*see* Appendix 15).

Sanfilippo syndrome: One of the mucopolysaccharidoses (type III) that is autosomal recessive and results in an accumulation of heparan sulfate. It is divided into 4 types based on their deficient enzyme: heparan N-sulfatase (type A); alpha-N-acetylglucosaminidase (type B); acetyl CoA:alpha-glucosaminide acetyltransferase (type C); and N-acetylglucosamine 6-sulfatase (type D). Patients may present with spasticity, motor dysfunction, hyperactivity, and developmental delay.

Chen AF, ed.
*Quick Reference Dictionary
for Orthopedics (pp 156-173).*
© 2012 Taylor & Francis Group.

Sangeorzan classification: A fracture classification system for navicular fractures in the foot (*see* Appendix 15).

sanguineous: Bloody fluid that has the same color as blood.

sarcoidosis: An inflammatory disease in which multiple granulomas form nodules in various organs, including skin, liver, lungs, spleen, eyes, joints, and muscles.

sarcoma: Malignant tissue that originates in connective tissue and spreads hematogenously.

Sarmiento brace: A functional brace used to immobilize midshaft humerus fractures (*see* Appendix 18).

sartorius: A muscle that flexes and externally rotates the hip. It originates from the anterior superior iliac spine (ASIS) and inserts into the proximal medial tibia (pes anserinus). It is Latin for tailor and it is the longest muscle in the body.

saucerization: A surgical procedure by which a cavity is created to expose the contents to the surface.

scaphoid: A carpal bone in the proximal row that looks like a boat and articulates with the lunate, capitate, trapezium, trapezoid, and radius. Also called the navicular bone of the hand. It is the most commonly fractured bone in the wrist.

scapula: Flattened, triangular bone that is part of the pectoral girdle connected to the clavicle and humerus. *Synonym*: Shoulder blade.

scapular winging: A physical exam finding where the scapula protrudes posteriorly due to loss of the long thoracic nerve (cervical nerve roots 5, 6, and 7) or paralysis of the serratus anterior muscle.

scapular Y view: A technique to capture radiographs of the scapular body and proximal humerus to evaluate for fractures. The patient is sitting up with the anterior affected shoulder on the x-ray cassette. The contralateral shoulder is 40 degrees off of the cassette. The beam is aimed from posterior to anterior along the scapular spine.

scapulopexy: Surgical fixation of the scapula to the chest wall. May be used to treat scapular winging.

Schanz pin: A specific type of threaded pin used in external fixators. Also known as a Schanz screw.

Schatzker classification: A fracture classification for tibia plateau fractures (*see* Appendix 15).

Scheuermann's disease: Abnormal wedging of 3 or more thoracic or thoracolumbar vertebrae and irregularities of the growth plate, which results in kyphosis. Also known as juvenile kyphosis.

Schmorl node: Vertical herniation of intervertebral discs into vertebral bodies, often found in degenerative spines. Best visualized with magnetic resonance imaging (MRI) or computed tomography (CT).

sciatica: Nerve inflammation along the L4 and L5 nerve root characterized by sharp pain along the sciatic nerve and its branches. This radiculopathy extends from the hip, down the back of the thigh, and distally to the remainder of the lower extremity.

sciatic nerve block: A regional delivery of local anesthetic agent that reduces pain and sensation in the distal leg (sciatic nerve distribution), except for the medial leg that is innervated by the saphenous nerve.

scissor dissection: A surgical maneuver that uses scissors to dissect through tissue.

scleroderma: A systemic autoimmune disease where the endothelial and smooth muscle cells are replaced by collagen and fibrous tissue. Patients often present with cutaneous manifestations of thickened and hardened skin on the arms and legs that results in limb contractures, especially seen in limited systemic scleroderma. Other organs, such as the lungs, esophagus, kidneys, and heart, are affected in diffuse systemic scleroderma.

sclerosing osteitis: Inflammation of bone in which areas become thickened and distended but no pus is formed. Also known as Garre disease.

sclerosis: Chronic swelling or inflammation of tissue that results in scarring.

scoliosis: Abnormal lateral curvature of the spine. This usually consists of 2 curves, the original abnormal curve and a compensatory curve in the opposite direction. Diagnosed by x-rays of the spine. Magnetic resonance imaging (MRI) may be warranted if there is rapid curve progression, neurological symptoms, or a left thoracic curve.

screening: Research process of examining a population for a given state or disease to determine whether they meet the inclusion criteria for a study.

scurvy: A disease due to lack of vitamin C that results in defective collagen formation. Patients present with poor wound healing, gum disease, and easy bruising.

segmental fracture: A fracture pattern where the long bone is broken in multiple pieces, where the midportion of bone is free from proximal and distal bone fragments.

segond fracture: An avulsion fracture of the lateral tibial condyle that is often associated with anterior cruciate ligament (ACL) tears and medial meniscus injury.

semimembranosus: A hamstring muscle that extends the hip and flexes the leg. It originates from the ischial tuberosity and inserts in the posterior medial tibial condyle.

semitendinosus: A hamstring muscle that extends the hip and flexes the leg that is often used as a graft for anterior cruciate ligament reconstruction. It originates from the ischial tuberosity and inserts in the pes anserinus.

sensation: Receiving conscious sensory impressions through direct stimulation of the body.

sensitivity: Statistical term describing the proportion of patients who test positive for a disease who truly have it. For tests that are highly sensitive, a negative result would rule out a disease.

sepsis: A life-threatening infection within the bloodstream due to released toxins. Patients often present with malaise, fevers, chills, low blood pressure, and mental status changes.

septic arthritis: An infection in a joint caused by bacteria.

septicemia: Systemic disease associated with the presence and persistence of pathogenic microorganisms or toxins in the blood.

septum: A structure that separates 2 areas of the body or 2 structures, often composed of a thin wall of tissue.

sequela: Morbid condition resulting from another condition or event.

sequential compression device (SCD): Intermittent pneumatic compression system that reduces the rate of deep vein thrombosis by activating blood flow. These are often used in nonambulatory patients or patients with limited mobility, especially during the postoperative period.

sequestrum: Fragment of necrosed bone that has become separated from the surrounding tissue.

serendipity view: A technique to capture radiographs of the sternoclavicular joint and medial one-third clavicle. The patient is supine with the cassette behind the upper chest, with the beam directed 40 degrees cephalad.

serial casting: Process of applying multiple casts of progressively changing positions to slowly bring a patient's limb to the desired position.

serosangineous: Body fluid that combines blood and serous fluid that is often pink tinged. Used to describe wound drainage that may be seen in the postoperative phase.

serous: Body fluid that resembles serum, or a yellow-colored, protein-rich fluid that separates when blood coagulates. Used to describe wound drainage that is commonly found in patients with excessive edema.

sesamoid: A small or oblong bone that is embedded in tendon that acts as a fulcrum for a tendon (the patella) or protects a tendon from direct pressure (the head of the first metatarsal bone).

sessile: Description of tissue where the attachment is a flat base.

Sever disease: A disease where the apophysis of the calcaneus is inflamed, which leads to pain with walking.

shaken baby syndrome: A form of child abuse where an infant is shaken. Clinical manifestation includes retinal hemorrhages and ecchymosis. May result in rib and long bone fractures.

sharp dissection: A surgical method of cutting through soft tissue using a sharp instrument, such as a scalpel.

shear: A force acting on an object in a perpendicular direction to the object that results in strain.

sheath: A smooth connective tissue sleeve that contains anatomical structures and allows for motion against surrounding structures.

Shenton line: An imaginary arch drawn from the inferior part of the femoral neck to the inferior border of the superior pubic ramus on an anteroposterior (AP) pelvis x-ray. A disruption of the Shenton line may indicate developmental dysplasia of the hip or a femoral neck fracture.

shin: A colloquial term for the tibia, which is the larger bone in the leg.

shin splints: Inflammation of the periosteum of the anterior tibia secondary to a rapid increase in activity.

shoe: An orthotic that provides a protective covering to the foot.

shoe lift: An insert placed into a shoe to add height to one leg in order to equalize leg lengths.

short arm cast (SAC): A cast that extends from below the elbow to proximal to the heads of the metacarpals that is molded in the interosseous membrane between the radius and the ulna (*see* Appendix 17).

short arm splint (SAS): A splint where plaster is applied to the volar surface of the forearm and secured with an elastic bandage (*see* Appendix 17).

short leg cast (SLC): A cast that extends from below the tibial tubercle to the heads of the metatarsals with ankle dorsiflexion to 90 degrees that is molded in the arch and Achilles tendon (*see* Appendix 17).

short leg splint (SLS): A splint where plaster is applied in 2 different orientations to secure fractures in the lower leg. One option is to apply plaster to the posterior leg from below the knee to beyond the toes, otherwise called a posterior splint. Another option is to apply plaster posteriorly below the knee and on the medial and lateral sides of the leg, otherwise called a team splint. Both are secured with elastic bandages and the ankle is dorsiflexed to 90 degrees (*see* Appendix 17).

shoulder: The joint formed by the articulation of the proximal humerus and the glenoid off of the scapula.

shoulderblade: A colloquial term for the scapula.

shoulder girdle: The bony arch that supports the arms, including the scapula, clavicle, and coracoid process. Also known as the pectoral girdle.

shunt: Passage between 2 channels, especially blood vessels, that may occur naturally or due to a disease process.

side effect: An outcome other than the desired action (eg, effect produced by a drug).

side pinch: A physical exam test where a pinch is performed using the side of a finger pressed against the thumb.

sinus tarsi: A sulcus between the inferior surface of the talus and superior surface of the calcaneus that travels over the lateral hindfoot and contains the interosseous talocalcaneal ligament. Also called the tarsal canal or talocalcaneal sulcus.

sinus tract: A pathway originating from an area in the body to the skin surface. An open channel by which bodily fluid may exit but that predisposes the patient to infection. Often occurs postoperatively in a nonhealing wound.

Sjögren syndrome: A systemic autoimmune disease where autoantibodies attack the exocrine glands, including the lacrimal and salivary glands. Patients often present with dry eyes and mouth, and may present with a spectrum of other autoimmune diseases.

skeletal system: Supporting framework for the body that is composed of the axial and appendicular divisions.

skilled nursing facility (SNF): Institution that provides care under the supervision of professional personnel, such as a registered nurse.

skin graft: A surgical procedure by which skin from one location is transferred to another location to provide wound coverage.

sling: An orthosis used to provide support to the proximal upper extremity.

slipped capital femoral epiphysis (SCFE): A fracture through the physis proximal to the femoral head that results in the femoral head (capital) sliding off of the femoral neck. This classically occurs in young, obese, and male patients.

slipped disc: A colloquial term for a herniated disc.

slough: Loose, stringy, necrotic tissue.

Sly syndrome: One of the mucopolysaccharidoses (type VII) in which there is a deficiency in beta-glucuronidase that results in the buildup of heparan and dermatan sulfate, as well as chondroitin 4,6-sulfate. Patients may present with skeletal dysplasia, short stature, hepatosplenomegaly, developmental delay, and corneal clouding.

Smith-Peterson approach: An anterior surgical approach to the hip through the internervous plane of the sartorius and tensor fascia lata, as well as the rectus femoris and gluteus medius.

Smith wrist fracture: Fracture of the distal radius with volar (or anterior) displacement of the hand. Often caused by a fall onto a flexed hand.

snapping hip syndrome: A medical condition in which there is a snapping sensation when the hip is flexed then extended. The causes may be extra-articular (iliotibial band/tensor fascia lata/gluteus medius rubbing against the greater trochanter with or without greater trochanteric bursitis) or intra-articular (torn acetabular labrum, ligamentum teres tear, loose bodies, or synovial chondromatosis). *Synonyms*: Coxa saltans, iliopsoas tendinitis, dancer's hip.

snuffbox: The anatomic region between the extensor pollicis longus and the abductor pollicis longus tendons that people use to sniff powered tobacco out of. Tenderness in this region may denote a scaphoid injury.

SOAP (subjective, objective, assessment, plan): The 4 parts of a written medical progress note, which includes the patient's state, a physical exam, an assessment of the patient, and the plan for patient care.

socket: (1) The hollow portion of a joint that contains the head of another bone. (2) The part of a prosthesis into which a stump of the remaining limb fits.

soft tissue: All neuromusculoskeletal tissues except bone and articular cartilage.

sole: A colloquial term for the plantar surface of the foot.

somatosensory evoked potential (SSEP): Peripheral nerve stimulation produces potentials that can be recorded from the scalp, over the spine, and/or from extremities.

spasm: An involuntary muscle contraction.

spastic: Muscle hyperactivity often from central nervous system disease that results in uncoordinated movements and contractures.

spastic diplegia: An increase in postural tone that is distributed primarily in the lower extremities and the pelvic area.

spastic gait: Walking characterized by stiff movements, slightly flexed hips and knee, dragging toes and adducted legs.

spasticity: Increase in muscle tone and stretch reflex of a muscle, resulting in increased resistance to passive stretch of the muscle and hyperresponsivity of the muscle to sensory stimulation.

spastic quadriplegia: An increase in postural tone in all 4 extremities, making it difficult to control posture.

specificity: Statistical term describing the proportion of patients who test negative for a disease and truly do not have it. For tests that are highly specific, a positive result would rule in a disease.

spicule: A sharp piece of bone or a pointed object.

spina bifida: A congenital disorder in which the embryonic neural tube fails to fully form and the 2 laminae fail to fuse. This leads to a spectrum of conditions where there is minimal clinical manifestation of disease (spina bifida occulta) to exposure of neural elements (myeloschisis, myelomeningocele).

spina bifida occulta: The most benign form of spina bifida where the posterior elements of vertebrae do not fully form but there is no protrusion of the spinal cord or meninges. Patients may present with a tuft of hair or skin changes overlying the defect.

spinal block: A local anesthetic administered inside the dura to reduce pain in a specific area. Often used when performing surgery in the lower extremities.

spinal canal: The bony structure that houses the spinal cord.

spinal cord: The portion of the nervous system that is found within the spinal canal that connects the brain to the remainder of the body.

spinal fusion: A surgical fusion of bone between 2 or more vertebrae that prevents movement that is used to stabilize the spine after fracture or surgical fixation.

spinal nerve: The nerve extending from the spinal cord.

spinal shock: Spinal shock usually involves a 24- to 72-hour period of paralysis, hypotonia, hyporeflexia or areflexia following a spinal cord injury (SCI), most often due to complete spinal cord transection. Return of reflex activity below the level of injury (such as the bulbocavernosus reflex) indicates the end of spinal shock. There can be bradycardia present in neurogenic shock, as opposed to tachycardia and hypotension with hypovolemic shock.

spinal stenosis: A narrowing of the spinal canal that causes compression of the spinal cord and nerve roots. Symptoms are usually referred into the buttocks and posterior thigh.

spine: (1) The 30 bony vertebrae that surround the spinal cord (7 cervical, 12 thoracic, 5 lumbar, 5 sacral, and 1 coccygeal). (2) Bony prominences found in the center of the tibial plateau.

spinocerebellar tracts: Dorsal tract consisting of the afferent ipsilateral ascending tract to the cerebellum, serving most lower extremities for touch, pressure, and proprioception. The ventral tract consisting of the afferent contralateral ascending tract to the cerebellum serves the lower extremities for proprioception.

spinothalamic tract (STT): Afferent contralateral and ipsilateral ascending tract to thalamus for sensation of pain, temperature, and light touch; also known as anterolateral system (ALS).

spiral fracture: A fracture pattern due to a twisting injury where the fracture travels from medial to lateral along a bone segment. Also called a torsion fracture.

spiral groove: A groove within the midshaft of the humerus bone where the radial nerve travels.

splint: Supportive device used to immobilize, fix, or prevent deformities or assist in motion. Support of a body segment through application of an external device (*see* Appendix 17).

split-thickness skin graft (STSG): An autograft technique used for wound coverage where the epidermis and part of the dermis is taken from another section of the body.

spondylitis: Inflammation of the vertebrae.

spondyloarthritis: Inflammatory joint disease, or arthritis, of the vertebrae.

spondylolisthesis: Subluxation of one vertebra over another, usually L5 anterior to the sacrum or L4 anterior to L5. Three main types include (1) isthmic, due to trauma; (2) degenerative, most common, patients generally over 50 years old, and presents with facet arthrosis; and (3) congenital.

spondylolysis: A defect of the pars interarticularis that most commonly occurs at L5.

spondylosis: Degenerative disease of the spine.

sprain: Injury to a joint that causes pain and disability, with the severity depending on the degree of injury to ligaments or tendons.

Sprengel deformity: A rare congenital abnormality in which the scapula does not decend, which results in an elevated and medially rotated scapula. May present with Klippel-Feil syndrome. Also known as congenital elevation of the scapula.

spring ligament: The plantar calcaneonavicular ligament that connects the sustentaculum tali of the calcaneus to the navicular that provides support to the medial longitudinal arch of the foot and to the head of the talus.

stack splint: A splint made of plastic that holds the distal phalanx in extension that is used to treat mallet finger.

stage: Classification of tumors by their metastases or spread throughout the body.

stance phase: One of the phases of gait that represents 60% of the gait cycle where the foot is touching the ground. It begins with heel strike and is followed by midstance, where the knee is extended and both feet touch the ground. It ends with terminal stance, where the foot is poised for toe-off.

standard deviation: Mathematically determined value used to derive standard scores and compare raw scores to a unit normal distribution.

standard error: Possible range in the variability of a person's "true" score in a test; a number that recognizes the amount by which a score may vary in different situation.

standard error of the mean: Standard deviation of an entire distribution of random sample means successively selected from a single population.

standardization: Method by which test scores of a typical population are derived, thus allowing subsequent test scores to be analyzed in light of that broad population; standardization requires a rigorous process of data collection and comparison.

standard score: Raw scores mathematically converted to a scale that facilitates comparison.

Staphylococcus aureus: A gram-positive bacteria that resides in the skin and is the most common organism found in orthopedic infections. This organism may be methicillin sensitive (MSSA) or methicillin resistant (MRSA). Traditionally, MSSA was acquired in the community and MRSA was acquired in the hospital setting, but current trends demonstrate that MRSA may be acquired in the community as well.

stapler: A device used to discharge staples that can be used to close wounds or organs.

stasis: Stagnant blood caused by venous congestion. Often occurs in the dependent lower extremities.

static splint: Rigid orthosis used for the prevention of movement of a joint or for the fixation of a displaced part.

Steinmann pin: A long pin with a sharp point used for fracture fixation or fracture stabilization using an external fixator. Can be smooth or threaded.

stellate fracture: A fracture pattern that resembles a star; often after direct trauma.

stenosis: A narrowing of any canal (eg, spinal stenosis with a narrowing of the spinal canal and intervertebral foramen).

sterile: For surgery, a condition in which an object is free of living organisms.

sterilization: The process by which living organisms are removed from materials, such as surgical instruments. Methods include gas, steam under pressure, and ionizing radiation.

sternoclavicular joint (SC joint): The joint in the trunk where the sternum articulates with the clavicle.

sternum: The bone in the front of the chest where the first 10 ribs attach.

steroid: An anti-inflammatory medication that binds to glucocorticoid receptors and upregulates anti-inflammatory molecules. Often used systemically or intraarticularly for treatment of arthritis.

Still disease: A form of juvenile rheumatoid arthritis where patients present with joint pain, fever, chills, and enlarged lymph nodes and spleen.

stinger: A contusion in the anterior part of the hip, often seen in football players. *Synonym:* Pointer.

stippled: In orthopedics, small, punctate calcifications in uncalcified regions of bone, such as cartilage. Often seen in infants and children.

stockinette: A woven cotton material that comes in the form of a tube that can be placed under casts. Impervious or permeable sterile stockinettes are also used in the operating room to cover an extremity while preparing the surgical field.

stocking glove distribution: A pattern of sensory loss due to peripheral neuropathy that follows the distribution of a stocking glove (distal arms and legs). Often seen in diabetic patients.

straight leg raise test: A physical exam finding that detects back pathology. The patient is placed supine on the examining table and one leg is raised with the knee in extension in order to stretch the sciatic nerve. If either leg exhibits pain, it is a sign of a herniated disc that is irritating the nerve root as it exits the spine. Also known as the Fajersztajn test or sciatic phenomenon.

strain: (1) The percentage change in original length of a deformed tissue. (2) A muscular injury caused by excessive physical effort that leads to a forcible stretch.

stress fracture: A break in the bone that produces a hairline fracture due to repetitive stress. May have to be diagnosed with magnetic resonance imaging (MRI).

strut graft: A graft made of cortical bone that gives structural support to bone.

Stryker notch view: A technique to capture radiographs of the humeral head, where the patient is supine on the table and the shoulder is forward flexed to 90 degrees. The beam is then directed 10 degrees proximally and centered over the coracoid process.

stump shrinker: An elastic sock that is applied to an amputated extremity to compress tissues prior to fitting for a prosthesis.

styloid process: A bony prominence at the end of bone, most notably at the distal ulna and distal radius.

subacromial bursitis: Inflammation of the bursa in the shoulder that is under the acromion and above the supraspinatus and infraspinatus (rotator cuff muscle). May be treated conservatively by activity modification, physical therapy, and corticosteroid injections or surgically with subacromial decompression.

subchondral bone: Dense bone below the surface of articular cartilage.

subcutaneous: The layer of fatty tissue that underlies the skin.

subcuticular suture: A stitch that is placed immediately below the skin, often in a running pattern.

sublingual (SL): Under the tongue.

subluxation: Partial or incomplete dislocation or movement away from an anatomical position (eg, shoulder, patella).

subscapularis: A muscle that internally rotates and adducts the arm. It originates from the subscapular fossa on the scapula and inserts into the lesser tuberosity.

subtalar arthrodesis: A fusion between the talus and calcaneus to correct back to anatomic alignment or for treating arthritis of the subtalar joint.

subtalar dislocation: Displacement of the talus or calcaneus from the talocalcaneal joint.

subtalar joint: The joint between the inferior talus and superior calcaneus.

subtrochanteric fracture: A fracture below the lesser trochanter of the femur that may require more distal fracture fixation.

subungual: The area beneath a nail.

suction: The application of negative pressure (air or water) to a system. Used in the operating room to clear fluid from the surgical field.

sugar tong splint: A splint that is applied to the forearm to immobilize the wrist and elbow. It is applied from proximal to the metacarpal heads on the volar surface of the hand, around the elbow, and to the dorsum of the hand (*see* Appendix 17).

sulcus: A fissure or groove in bone or tissue.

sundowning: Condition in which persons tend to become more confused or disoriented at the end of the day. May be exacerbated in the postoperative state.

sunrise view: An x-ray view of the patella where the x-ray beam is tangential to the patella to view the patealla within the femoral sulcus of the distal femur.

superficial: Area of the body that is located closes to the surface.

superficial vein thrombosis (SVT): A blood clot in a superficial vein of the extremities that often presents with induration, pain, and localized erythema.

superior: (1) In anatomical position, located above. (2) Toward the head or upper portion of a part or structure. *Synonym*: Cephalad.

superior gemellus: A muscle that is a short external rotator of the hip. It originates from the ischial spine and inserts in the medial greater trochanter.

superior labrum anterior and posterior (SLAP) tear: A tear of the superior labrum of the shoulder that is often treated with arthroscopic surgery.

supination: The act of assuming the supine position. (1) Rotation of the forearm outward (laterally) so that the palm is facing toward the ceiling. (2) For the foot, turning the plantar surface of the foot inward. Involves a combination of inversion and adduction to raise the longitudinal arch of the foot.

supinator: A muscle that supinates the forearm. It originates on the posterior medial ulna and inserts in the proximal lateral radius.

supine: Lying on the spine with the face up.

suppression: The ability of the central nervous system to screen out certain stimuli so that others may be attended to more carefully.

suppuration: The formation and discharge of pus.

suppurative: A type of infection that exudes pus.

supracondylar fracture: A type of fracture pattern in the condyles of the distal femur and distal humerus.

suprapatellar pouch: The synovial lined cavity superior to the patella that is the proximal portion of the knee joint. Often the first location viewed during a knee arthroscopy.

supraspinatus: One of the rotator cuff muscles that initiates abduction of the arm. It originates in the supraspinatus fossa of the scapula and inserts into the greater tuberosity.

supraspinatus outlet view: A technique to capture radiographs of the supraspinatus and coracoacromial arches. The patient is sitting up with the anterior affected shoulder on the x-ray cassette. The contralateral shoulder is 40 degrees off of the cassette. The beam is aimed from posterior to anterior along the scapular spine with a 10-degree caudal tilt.

surgical neck fracture: A fracture of the proximal humerus below the physeal plate.

sustentaculum tali: The portion of bone in the medial calcaneus that supports the talus. Multiple ligaments attach there, including the spring ligament, tibiocalcaneal ligament, and medial talocalcaneal ligament. Also known as a talar shelf.

suture: The material used to close a wound that may be absorbable (gut) or not absorbable (silk or nylon).

suture anchor: A surgical implant where a screw is attached to sutures with or without needles. The screw is fixed into bone, and the sutures are used to repair tendons or ligaments to the bone.

swan neck deformity: Condition of the hand characterized by hyperextension of the proximal interphalangeal joint and flexion of the distal interphalangeal joint. Often found in patients with rheumatoid arthritis and Ehlers-Danlos syndrome.

swing phase: One of the phases of gait that represents 40% of the gait cycle where the foot is not touching the ground. It is further divided into preswing, initial swing, mid-swing, and terminal swing.

Symes amputation: A surgical removal of the foot through the tibiotalar joint, where the heel pad is covers the distal surface of the tibia.

sympathetic nervous system: Autonomic nervous system that mobilizes the body's resources during stressful situations.

symphysis: Articulation of 2 bones connected by cartilage that do not move (eg, pubic symphysis).

synarthrosis: A joint where there is little to no movement, often due to a fibrous tissue connection.

syndactyly: Webbing of the fingers (or toes) involving only the skin or, in complex cases, the fusing of adjacent bones. Mostly seen in children.

syndesmosis: Articulation between bones formed by interosseous ligaments (eg, tibia and fibula).

syndrome: Combination of symptoms resulting from a single course or commonly occurring together that they constitute a distinct clinical picture.

synergy: Muscles that work together to produce a desired effect.

synostosis: Fusion between 2 bones (not through a joint).

synovectomy: Excision of the synovial membrane.

synovial chondromatosis: Numerous small cartilaginous formations in synovium that become loose bodies within a joint. Often found in the knee, hip, or elbow and causes a great deal of pain and decreased range of motion.

synovial fluid: A viscous substance produced by the synovium in joints that reduces friction between the articular surfaces of cartilage and lubricates joints. It is composed of hyaluronic acid, lubricin, collagenases, and proteinases.

synovial sarcoma: A rare malignant soft tissue tumor that commonly arises around large joints. It often affects the SSX1-SYT genes and contains the t(X;18) translocation. Cells stain positive with keratin and epithelial membrane antigen (EMA), and histology demonstrates a biphasic cell distribution with epithelial cells alternating with spindle cells.

synovitis: Inflammation of the synovium.

synovium: A soft tissue membrane that lines the noncartilaginous portions of a joint and produces synovial fluid.

syringomyelia: Chronic progressive degeneration disorder of the spinal cord characterized by the development of an irregular cavity within the spinal cord.

systemic: Affecting the entire body.

tabes dorsalis: A neurologic sequelae of late syphilis, where there is a loss of sensation and position sense in the lower extremities. Also known as posterior spinal sclerosis.

tachycardia: Rapid heartbeat (above 100 beats per minute).

tachypnea: Rapid respirations marked by quick, shallow breathing (respiratory rate above 20).

tailbone: A colloquial term for the coccyx.

talipes: Deformities of the foot, especially those congenital in origin. *Synonym*: Clubfoot.

talocalcaneal bar: A congenital bridge of bone formed between the talus and calcaneus that limits subtalar motion.

tamponade: The process by which increased pressure prevents blood or fluid to enter an area.

tantalum metal: A transition metal that is resistant to corrosion. Used in some orthopedic implants.

tapered needle: A type of needle used in suturing with a blunted tip to burrow through tissue when it is passed.

tarsal bones: The hindfoot, consisting of the talus, calcaneus, navicular, cuboid, and 3 cuneiforms. These correlate with the 8 carpal bones in the hand.

tarsometatarsal (TMT): The joint between the tarsal and metatarsal bones of the foot.

Tay Sachs disease: An autosomal recessive disorder caused by a genetic defect in chromosome 15 that results in deficiency of hexosaminidase A and an accumulation of gangliosides. Patients present with progressive spastic paralysis, cherry red maculas, blindness, and mental retardation.

T-condylar fracture: A fracture pattern in the supracondylar region of the humerus where there is a transverse component and a vertical component that divides the medial and lateral condyles, which resembles the letter T on x-ray.

Chen AF, ed.
*Quick Reference Dictionary
for Orthopedics (pp 174-183).*

Technetium-99: The radioactive material injected into the blood stream for a bone scan.

TED stockings: (Covidien, Mansfield, Massachusetts) A trademark name for anti-thromboembolic stockings to prevent deep vein thromboses (DVTs).

Telfa dressing: A dressing covered in a plastic material that does not stick to wounds.

tendinitis: Inflammation of tendons, often at the insertion point into bone.

tendoachilles: The tendon that connects the triceps surae to the calcaneus that is composed of the gastrocnemius and soleus tendons. This muscle is often lengthened or released in pediatric patients with clubfeet and is often ruptured in middle-aged males while playing sports. *Synonyms*: Achilles tendon, heel cord.

tendon: Structure composed of strong, fibrous tissue that attaches muscles to bones.

tennis elbow: Lateral epicondylitis; or inflammation and focal hyaline degeneration of the extensor carpi radialis brevis (ECRB) or extensor digitorum communis (EDC).

tenodesis: Surgical fixation of a tendon.

tenolysis: Surgical separation of a tendon from adhesions.

tenosynovectomy: The surgical removal of the inflamed lining of tendons.

tenosynovitis: The inflammation of the lining overlying a tendon.

tenotomy: Surgical cutting of a tendon.

tensile force: Resistive force generated with a tissue in response to elongation or stretch.

tensor fascia latae: A muscle that abducts, flexes, and internally rotates the thigh. It originates from the anterior superior iliac spine (ASIS) and iliac crest and inserts into the iliotibial band.

teres major: A muscle that internally rotates and adducts the arm. It originates from the inferior angle of the scapula and inserts into the intertubercular groove in the humerus.

teres minor: One of the rotator cuff muscles that externally rotates the arm. It originates from the lateral scapula and inserts into the greater tuberosity.

test protocol: Specific procedures that must be followed when assessing a patient; formal testing procedures.

tethered cord syndrome: A condition in children where the conus medullaris, or the terminal end of the spinal cord, is attached to scar tissue or bone. This prevents the spinal cord from migrating upward as the patient grows. Increased cord tension may cause progressive lower extremity paralysis and changes in bowel or bladder function.

tetraplegia: Impairment or loss of motor and/or sensory function in the cervical spinal cord that affects all 4 limbs. *Synonym*: Quadriplegia.

thenar atrophy: Loss of muscle mass in the thenar eminence, due to disease (eg, carpal tunnel syndrome) or disuse.

thenar eminence: The musculature of the thumb, consisting of the abductor pollicis brevis (APB), opponens pollicis, and adductor pollicis (oblique head).

thigh: The area containing the anatomical structures between the hip and the knee.

thighbone: A colloquial term for the femur.

Thomas test: A physical exam test to look for hip flexion contractures by evaluating the iliopsoas muscle. The patient is placed supine on the examining table, one leg is flexed to his or her chest, and the other leg is extended. If the hip remains flexed or too much pain occurs during extension, then the patient has tight hip flexors.

Thompson and Epstein classification: A classification system for posterior hip dislocations (*see* Appendix 15).

thoracic: Pertaining to or situated near the chest.

thoracic spine: The portion of the spine between the cervical and lumbar spines consisting of 12 vertebrae that provides support for the ribs.

thoracolumbar: The areas of the spine that include the thoracic and lumbar regions.

thorax: The chest, or the part of the body between the neck and the abdomen that is delineated by the thoracic spinal vertebrae and the 12 ribs attached to them.

threshold: Level at which a stimulus is recognized by sensory receptors.

thrombin: The enzyme derived from prothrombin that converts fibrinogen to fibrin; part of the common coagulation cascade.

thrombocytopenia: A condition in which the blood platelets are destroyed, causing severe bleeding if injury occurs.

thrombolytic: Dissolving or splitting up a thrombus, either mechanically or chemically.

thrombophlebitis: Inflammation of a vein associated with thrombus formation.

thrombosis: Coagulation of the blood to form a clot locally, especially in the heart or blood vessels.

thrombus: A locally formed blood clot within the circulatory system.

thumb spica cast: A cast that extends from below the elbow to proximal to the heads of the metacarpals that also immobilizes the thumb in abduction past the interphalangeal joint. It is given an interosseous mold between the radius and ulna (*see* Appendix 17).

thumb spica splint: A splint where plaster is applied along the thumb and down the radial side of the forearm to below the elbow and secured with an elastic bandage. The thumb is immobilized past the interphalangeal joint (*see* Appendix 17).

tibialis anterior: A muscle in the anterior compartment of the leg that dorsiflexes and inverts the foot. It originates from the lateral tibia and interosseous membrane and inserts in the base of the first metatarsal and medial cuneiform.

tibialis posterior: A muscle in the posterior compartment of the leg that plantarflexes and inverts the foot. It originates from the posterior interosseous membrane and inserts in the navicular, cuneiform, and metatarsals.

tibial torsion: Rotation occurring inherently in the shaft of the tibia from the proximal to distal ends.

Tillaux fracture: A pattern where the anterolateral articular surface of the distal tibia is fractured.

Tinel sign: A physical exam finding where tapping the area overlying an irritated nerve (due to injury, compression, or regeneration) results in a tingling or shocking sensation down the distribution of that nerve.

thoracolumbosacral orthosis (TLSO): A brace used to immobilize the thoracic, lumbar, and sacral spines, either after a fracture, postsurgically, or to correct scoliosis (*see* Appendix 18).

Tommy John procedure: A reconstruction of the ulnar collateral ligament at the elbow, which was made famous by the pitcher Tommy John in 1974.

tone: State of muscle contraction at rest; may be determined by resistance to stretch.

tonnis angle: A radiographic angle to assess acetabular dysplasia, determined by drawing a horizontal line from the middle of the weight bearing portion of the acetabulum and a second line from this middle point to the lateral edge of the acetabulum. A normal measurement is less than 10 degrees; greater than 10 degrees is indicative of acetabular dysplasia.

tophus: A deposit of uric acid crystals commonly found in the first toe and ears as a result of gout.

torque: Rotating tendency of force; equals the produce of force and the perpendicular distance from the axis of a lever to the point of application of the same force.

torsion: A twisting force applied around an axis.

torticollis: A type of cervical dystonia where there is abnormal muscle spasm and tension of the sternocleidomastoid muscle innervated by the spinal accessory nerve that results in the head being fixed in one direction.

torus fracture: A break in the bone involving one cortex but not disrupting both cortices. *Synonym*: Buckle fracture.

total contact cast: A special cast constructed of plaster or fiberglass that is made to conform to the entire lower extremity. Mostly used to treat Charcot arthropathy and foot ulcers in diabetic patients.

total elbow arthroplasty (TEA): Replacing the distal humerus and proximal ulna with metal and plastic to create another joint to enable painless range of motion.

total hip arthroplasty (THA): A total hip replacement where the femoral head is removed and replaced with a metal stem and the acetabulum is reamed and replaced with a metal cup. The articulating surface ranges from polyethylene, ceramic, or metal.

total joint arthroplasty (TJA): Hip or knee replacements, where the entire surface of the articulating bones is replaced with artificial components.

total knee arthroplasty (TKA): A total knee replacement where the distal femur and proximal tibia are replaced by metal implants with an articulating polyethylene piece.

total parenteral nutrition (TPN): A method to provide nutrients to patients intravenously, without requiring oral intake.

total shoulder arthroplasty: A replacement of the humeral head with a stemmed prosthesis and of the glenoid to decrease pain within an arthritic joint. For patients with arthritis and rotator cuff pathology, the reverse total shoulder is performed.

touch down weight bearing (TDWB): A restriction in activity where a patient can only touch his or her toe to the ground to limit the weight transmitted through that extremity. Also known as toe touch weight bearing (TTWB).

tourniquet: A device that consists of a cuff that is inflated to apply pressure to an artery that decreases or stops blood flow to an extremity. Often used in surgery to minimize blood in the operative field and to minimize blood loss from an extremity.

trabecular: A substance with fine spicules that form a honeycomb appearance, often referring to bone.

trabecular metal: A material made of tantalum metal that resembles the structure of bone and is designed to improve bony ingrowth.

tract: A long path, often used to describe the path of nerve fibers that travel from the brain through the spinal cord.

traction: The therapeutic use of manual or mechanical tension created by a pulling force to produce a combination of distraction and gliding to relieve pain and increase tissue flexibility.

traction bed: A bed that is equipped with a distal attachment from which traction can be hung.

traction bow: A bow placed on either end of a wire embedded in bone that is used to pull traction on an extremity. Often applied to the proximal tibia or distal femur for pulling a midshaft femur fracture or acetabular fracture to length.

transcutaneous electrical nerve stimulation (TENS): Application of mild electrical stimulation to skin electrodes placed over the region of pain to cause interference with the transmission of painful stimuli.

transection: A surgical procedure in which a structure is cut.

transplant: A surgical procedure in which one part of a human body is moved to another part. It may be taken from oneself (eg, skin graft) or from a donor (eg, organ transplant).

transudate: A fluid substance that has passed through a membrane or has been extruded from a tissue, sometimes as a result of inflammation. A transudate, in contrast to an exudate, is characterized by low protein.

transverse: Across, vertical, or perpendicular to the long axis of the body.

transverse acetabular ligament: A ligament that is part of the acetabular labrum that marks the inferior border of the acetabulum. May be used as a landmark during hip surgery.

trapeze frame: An orthopedic device where metal struts are attached above the bed and handles are added to facilitate patient movement.

trapezius: A muscle that elevates and rotates the scapula. It originates from C7 to T12 spinous processes and inserts into the clavicle and acromion spine of the scapula. May lead to lateral winging of the scapula if the spinal accessory nerve is compromised.

trauma: Injury due to physical harm.

traumatic brain injury (TBI): Injury caused by impact to the head. An insult to the brain caused by an external physical force that may produce a diminished or altered state of consciousness, which results in impairment of cognitive abilities or physical functioning.

tremor: Involuntary shaking or trembling.

Trendelenburg gait: A gait that results from hip abductor weakness where the pelvis tilts to the opposite side and the patient lurches to the affected side to compensate.

Trendelenburg position: A position with the patient supine on a table with his or her feet higher than the head.

Trendelenburg sign: A physical exam finding where a patient stands on the leg of the side with weak hip abductor muscles and the pelvis drops toward the contralateral side.

triangles: Radiolucent metal frames shaped as triangles that are used to flex the knee at varying angles. Often used for placing intramedullary rods in the tibia for fracture fixation.

triangular fibrocartilage complex (TFCC): A triangular-shaped articular disk that is the major ligamentous stabilizer of the distal radioulnar joint (DRUJ) and ulnar carpus.

triceps brachii: A muscle composed of 3 heads that extends the forearm. The long head originates from the infraglenoid tubercle, the lateral head originates from the posterior proximal humerus, and the medial head originates from the posterior distal humerus. All insert in the proximal olecranon.

trigger finger: A pathological condition in which a finger catches when going from flexion to extension. Most commonly due to thickening or nodule formation within the A1 pulley. May be treated with corticosteroid injections or surgical release.

trigger points: Specific areas of the body that are tender when palpated. Commonly seen in fibromyalgia.

trimalleolar: The 3 prominences of bone in the ankle, specifically, the medial malleolus (tibia), lateral malleolus (fibula), and posterior malleolus (tibia).

triple arthrodesis: A surgical fusion of 3 joints within the ankle, including the talocalcaneal, talonavicular, and calcaneocuboid joints.

triradiate cartilage: The cartilaginous area in the acetabulum of an infant where the iliac, ischium, and pubis meet. These eventually fuse at age 14 to 16.

trocar: A surgical instrument with a sleeve or cannula covering a pointed pin. The pin is used to penetrate tissue and guide the blunter tool to a specific location.

trochanter: A prominence on the proximal femur, consisting of the greater trochanter (larger, lateral, and more proximal) and the lesser trochanter (smaller, medial, and more distal).

trochlea: A groove on bone where another bone articulates. Refers to the distal femur where the patella articulates or the distal humerus where the ulna articulates.

trophic: Changes that occur as a result of inadequate circulation, such as loss of hair, thinning of skin, and ridging of nails.

trunnion: A cylindrical protrusion that serves as a pivoting point. In total hip replacements, it refers to the proximal portion of the stem (neck) on which the head is mounted.

Tscherne classification: A classification system for soft tissue injury in closed fractures (*see* Appendix 15).

t Test: Parametric statistical test comparing differences of 2 data sets.

tubercle: Protrusion on a bone (eg, tibial tubercle).

tuberosity: A bony protuberance that is often the site of muscle or ligament attachments.

tuft: With regards to orthopedic bony anatomy, the distal portion of the distal phalanx of a finger or a toe.

tumor: Abnormal and unregulated growth of tissue that may be benign or malignant. Also called a neoplasm.

tunnel view: A radiographic view of the wrist to view the carpal tunnel or of the knee to view the intercondylar femoral notch (location of anterior and posterior cruciate ligaments).

turgid: Distended and swollen.

Turner syndrome: A chromosomal abnormality where females only have one X chromosome instead of 2, which results in shortened stature, shortened fourth metatarsals and metacarpals, osteoporosis, scoliosis, amenorrhea, aortic dilation, and neck webbing.

twisted neck: A colloquial term for torticollis.

two-tailed (nondirectional) test: A statistical test of the null hypothesis in which both tails of the distribution are utilized.

ulcer: An open sore on the skin or some mucous membrane characterized by the disintegration of tissue and often the discharge of serous drainage.

ulnar claw: A physical exam finding of the hand where the ring and small fingers are flexed at the proximal and distal interphalangeal joints, often due to a lesion of the ulnar nerve.

ulnar collateral ligament: (1) The connective tissue band that traverses the medial side of the elbow and connects the humerus and ulna. (2) The fibrous tissue band that connects the metacarpal to the proximal phalanx on the ulnar side of the digit.

ulnar deviation: Deviation toward the ulna, or the smaller of the 2 bones in the forearm. Also called ulnar drift.

ulnar gutter cast: A cast that extends from below the elbow to the tips of the ring and small fingers that treats ulnar fractures or boxers fractures. It is given an interosseous mold between the radius and ulna (*see* Appendix 17).

ulnar gutter splint: A splint where plaster is applied along the ring and small fingers and down the ulnar side of the forearm to below the elbow and secured with an elastic bandage. The ring and small fingers are immobilized past the distal interphalangeal joint (*see* Appendix 17).

ulnar negative variance: A variance in wrist anatomy where the ulna is shorter than the radius.

ulnar positive variance: A variance in wrist anatomy where the ulna is longer than the radius.

ultrasound (US): A diagnostic tool that uses high-frequency sound waves to produce images based on the echogenicity of a structure. Doppler US can be used to measure blood flow. US may also be used for therapeutic treatment, because the high-frequency sound waves generate heat. Also called high-intensity focused ultrasound (HIFU).

uncemented: A technique in arthroplasty where implants with porous and rough surfaces are press-fit into bone, which allows bone to grow into the implant and provide stable fixation.

undermine: Tissue destruction underlying intact skin along wound margins.

undifferentiated pleomorphic sarcoma: The more current name for malignant fibrous histiocytoma (MFH) that is a malignant soft tissue sarcoma with frequent metastases. *Synonym*: Pleomorphic undifferentiated sarcoma.

unhappy triad: An injury to the knee often sustained from a football tackle to the knees (clipping) that results in tears of the medial meniscus, medial collateral ligament (MCL), and anterior cruciate ligament (ACL).

unicameral bone cyst (UBC): A benign, well-defined, membrane-lined cavity that is filled with fluid; often found in children. They mostly occur near growth plates and are often found in a central location in bone. Also known as a simple bone cyst.

unicompartmental knee arthroplasty: A partial knee replacement where a prosthesis is used to replace either the medial or lateral side of the knee.

unilateral: Pertaining to one side.

union: Healing of a fracture or osteotomy site.

unipolar hemiarthroplasty: A prosthesis with no modularity and only one articulation between the head and socket. In hips, the head of the implant articulates with the native acetabulum. In shoulders, the head of the implant articulates with the native glenoid.

universal precautions: An approach to infection control designed to prevent transmission of blood-borne diseases, such as autoimmune deficiency syndrome (AIDS) and hepatitis B; includes specific recommendations for the use of gloves, protective eye wear, and masks.

University of California Berkley Laboratory (UCBL) orthosis: An arch support that is molded to the foot designed to passively correct hindfoot or forefoot abnormalities in order to treat flexible flatfoot deformity (*see* Appendix 18).

Unna boot: A compression dressing with gel, made primarily of zinc oxide, and gauze that is used to treat skin ulcers and to reduce swelling.

upper motor neuron (UMN): Neurons of the cerebral cortex that conduct stimuli from the motor cortex of the brain to motor nuclei of cerebral nerves of the ventral gray columns of the spinal cord.

upper motor neuron (UMN) disease: A disease of the neurons in the cerebral cortex where patients often present with hyperreflexia and spasticity.

urinalysis (UA): A laboratory test of urine to assess its contents that may be indicative of systemic disease.

vacuum-assisted closure (VAC) dressing: A type of negative pressure dressing that is applied to a wound using an airtight seal and attached to continuous or intermittent suction. This dressing draws out fluid and is able to increase the speed of granulation tissue formation.

valgus: A limb deformity where the extremity is moved away (ie, laterally) from the midline.

validity: Statistical term indicating the degree to which a test measures what it is intended to measure.

Van Nes rotationplasty: A type of surgical procedure used to treat congenital short femur or a femur deficiency by performing a tibial osteotomy and rotating the leg so that the ankle serves as a knee joint. A prosthesis can then be fitted to the foot so that the patient can ambulate.

variance: Statistical measurement that demonstrates how scores in a distribution deviate from the mean.

varus: A limb deformity where the extremity is moved toward (ie, medially) toward the midline.

vastus intermedius: The middle muscle of the quadriceps that extends the knee. It originates in the proximal femoral shaft and inserts in the patella.

vastus lateralis: The lateral muscle of the quadriceps that extends the knee. The muscle originates from the greater trochanter and inserts into the lateral patella.

vastus medialis: The most medial muscle of the quadriceps that extends the knee. The muscle originates from the intertrochanteric line (medial linea aspera) and inserts in the medial patella.

VATER syndrome: A constellation of congenital abnormalities that affect the following anatomic regions: vertebral, anus, trachea, esophagus, and renal. These patients may present with lumbosacral agenesis, anal imperforation, tracheoesophageal fistulas (TE), and renal agenesis.

Chen AF, ed.
*Quick Reference Dictionary
for Orthopedics* (pp 187-189).

vein: A vessel that carries deoxygenated blood to the heart, with the exception of the pulmonary vein, which carries oxygenated blood toward the heart from the lungs.

ventral: Anatomic position located toward the front of the body or toward the abdomen. *Synonym*: Anterior.

vertebra: One of the bones of the spine.

vertebroplasty: A surgical method for treating vertebral fractures where a needle is percutaneously inserted into a collapsed or fractured vertebra and bone cement is injected to stabilize the fracture and strengthen the weakened bone. This contrasts with kyphoplasty, in that a balloon is not used.

villous synovitis: Inflammation of the synovium that produces finger-like projections into a joint that hypertrophy with chronic irritation.

vinculum: A connective band of tissue that holds tendon to bone.

viscosupplementation: An intraarticular injection of hyaluronic acid that helps cushion the joint and decreases pain associated with osteoarthritis.

Visual Analog Scale (VAS): A tool used to objectively describe pain that allows a patient to indicate his or her degree of pain by pointing to a visual representation of pain intensity. The scale is usually 1 to 10 or 1 to 100, with the higher numbers representing greater pain.

vital signs: Measurements of pulse rate, respiration rate, body temperature, blood pressure, and oxygen saturation.

volar: Palm of the hand and anterior aspect of the forearm. *Synonym*: Anterior. *Antonym*: Dorsal.

volar dorsal splint: A splint made of plaster on the volar and doral surfaces of the forearm that runs from the proximal third of the forearm to the distal tips of the fingers with the wrist extended, the metacarpophalangeal joint flexed, and the interphalangeal joints extended. Secured with an elastic bandage (*see* Appendix 17).

volar splint: A splint made of plaster and secured with an elastic bandage that runs from the proximal third of the forearm to the distal tips of the fingers with the wrist extended and the metacarpophalangeal joint flexed (*see* Appendix 17).

Volkmann canals: The passages that connect osteons within bone.

Volkmann contracture: Permanent contracture of a muscle due to replacement of muscle with fibrous tissue that lacks the ability to contract. Often occurs after a missed compartment syndrome.

von Recklinghausen disease: The most common neurofibromatosis disease due to a mutation in neurofibromin on chromosome 17. Patients present with café au lait spots, harmatomas of the iris (Lisch nodules), optic glioma, and multiple neurofibromas. *Synonym*: Neurofibromatosis type I.

VY-plasty: A surgical procedure to lengthen tissue where a V-shaped incision is made in the middle of the skin flap, the tissue is advanced, and the incision is closed to look more like a Y. This type of closure is effective over fingertip amputations.

wake-up test: A clinical test where the patient is partially awakened or weaned from sedation so that a motor and sensory exam can be performed to assess the extent of spinal cord injury.

Wallerian degeneration: The physical and biochemical changes that occur in a nerve because of the loss of axonal continuity following trauma.

Ward triangle: An area of diminished density in the trabeculae of the femoral neck seen by x-ray and direct inspection of a specimen.

Watson-Jones approach: An anterolateral surgical approach to the hip utilizing the intermuscular plane between the gluteus medius and the tensor fascia lata.

Weber fracture: A fracture classification system for the lateral malleolus of the fibula based on the location of the fracture in relation to the joint (*see* Appendix 15).

Webril: (Covidien, Mansfield, Massachusetts) A trademark name for a specific cotton used in casting and splinting that is dense, soft, and easy to tear. This cotton permits swelling to occur and is used to pad bony prominences.

web space: The skin bridge that connects 2 digits (fingers or toes).

wedge fracture: A vertebral body fracture where the anterior or lateral edge is compressed.

wedging: A method of correcting the alignment of a cast that is accomplished by cutting the cast in a specific location and wedging the cast open to change the direction of the cast.

weightbearing: The amount of force that may be placed through a specified extremity.

weight bearing as tolerated (WBAT): An activity order where there is no restriction in activity.

Chen AF, ed.
*Quick Reference Dictionary
for Orthopedics* (pp 190-192).
© 2012 Taylor & Francis Group

weight bearing surface: The surface of a joint through which the load of the body travels.

West Point view: A technique to capture radiographs of the glenoid rim, where the patient is prone on the table and the arm is abducted and placed over an 8-cm pad. The beam is then directed 25 degrees toward the head and 25 degrees toward the midline of the body.

whiplash injury: Injury caused by sudden hyperextension and flexion of the neck, traumatizing cervical ligaments; common in rear-end car accidents or falls.

white blood cells (WBCs): Cells found in the immune system that defend against infection and foreign objects. Several types of WBCs are present within the immune system, including neutrophils, eosinophils, basophils, monocytes, macrophages, dendritic cells, and lymphocytes. Levels will be elevated in infection, except in immunocompromised patients. Also known as leukocytes.

white matter: Area of the central nervous system that contains the axons of the cells.

windshield wiper sign: A radiographic sign indicative of implant loosening in total joint arthroplasty where there is radiolucency around the stem of implants that occurs in the pattern that windshield wipers make.

windswept knees: A condition in which one knee is in valgus (knock-knee) and the other is in varus (bow-legged), making it look like the legs are being swept by the wind from the valgus side.

winging scapula: Medial or lateral protrusion of the scapula due to injury to the long thoracic nerve (serratus anterior muscle) or the spinal accessory (trapezius muscle) nerve, respectively.

Winquist and Hansen classification: A fracture classification system for femoral shaft fractures based on the degree of comminution (*see* Appendix 15).

within normal limits (WNL): Findings that are consistent with a normal physiologic state.

Wolff's law: A principle that states that bone is formed in areas of stress and resorbed in areas of no stress.

wound: An area of disrupted or discontinuous skin or tissue.

wound care: Procedures used to achieve a clean wound bed, promote a moist environment, facilitate autolytic debridement, or absorb excessive fluid exudate from a wound.

wound repair: Healing process of an open area of skin or tissue. Partial thickness involves epithelialization; full thickness involves contraction granulation and epithelialization. Consists of 3 phases: inflammatory, proliferative, and regenerative.

woven bone: A type of immature bone in areas of new growth, such as fracture healing or embryologic development. Osteoblasts produce osteoid rapidly, which results in disorganized collagen fibers that are mechanically weak. This bone is later replaced with lamellar bone.

Wrisberg ligament: The posterior meniscofemoral ligament, or the ligament that connects the posterior horn of the lateral meniscus to the medial femoral condyle.

wrist: The articulating joints between the carpal bones and radius and ulna.

xanthoma: An accumulation of fatty deposits in tendons and skin found in patients with high cholesterol levels.

xenograft: Transplantation of a biological sample obtained from another source of a different species (eg, tendons taken from a cow).

Xeroform: (Covidien, Mansfield, Massachusetts) A trademark yellow gauze that is used to dress wounds that contains petroleum and an antiseptic solution.

x-linked recessive: Trait transmitted by a gene located on the X chromosome. These traits are passed on by a carrier mother to an affected son. An example is Duchenne's muscular dystrophy.

x-ray: An imaging modality that uses ionizing radiation to image bones (*see* Appendix 22).

Young and Burgess classification: A fracture classification system for pelvic fractures based on the mechanism of injury (lateral compression or anterior posterior compression) (*see* Appendix 15).

y-plasty: A surgical procedure by which an incision is made in the shape of a Y in order to reshape a scar.

Z

Zanca view: A technique to capture radiographs of the acromioclavicular (AC) joint. The patient is seated and the beam is directed 10 to 15 degrees toward the head at the AC joint. The amount of x-ray penetration should be decreased so that the AC joint is not overexposed.

z-plasty: A surgical procedure by which multiple incisions are made in a zigzag pattern in order to reshape a scar or lengthen a tendon.

z score (standard score): (1) Numerical value from the transformation of a raw score into units of standard deviation. (2) A measurement of bone mineral density that compares a patient's bone density to the average values of a person of the same age and gender.

Bibliography

American Academy of Orthopaedic Surgeons. *Electro-diagnostic Testing*. Chicago, IL: American Academy of Orthopaedic Surgeons; 2007.

Bernier JN. *Quick Reference Dictionary for Athletic Training*. 2nd ed. Thorofare, NJ: SLACK Incorporated; 2005.

Bottomley JM. *Quick Reference Dictionary for Physical Therapy*. 2nd ed. Thorofare, NJ: SLACK Incorporated; 2003.

Editors of The American Heritage Dictionaries. *The American Heritage Dictionary*. 5th ed. Boston, MA: Houghton Mifflin Harcourt; 2011.

Egol KA, Koval KJ, Zuckerman JD. *Handbook of Fractures*. 4th ed. Philadelphia, PA: Lippincott Williams & Wilkins; 2010.

Gonzalez J, Bernstein S, Collins D. *Dictionary of Orthopedic Terminology*. Gainesville, FL: Triad Publishing Company; 2008.

Greenspan A. *Orthopedic Imaging: A Practical Approach*. 4th ed. Philadelphia, PA: Lippincott Williams & Wilkins; 2004.

Mollon B, da Silva V, Busse JW, Einhorn TA, Bhandari M. Electrical stimulation for long-bone fracture-healing: a meta-analysis of randomized controlled trials. *J Bone Joint Surg Am*. 2008;90:2322-2330.

Parvizi J, Klatt B. *Essentials in Total Knee Arthroplasty*. Thorofare, NJ: SLACK Incorporated; 2011.

PDR Staff. *Physicians' Desk Reference*. 65th ed. Montvale, NJ: PDR Network; 2011.

Rüedi TP, Buckley RE, Moran CG. *AO Principles of Fractures Management*. 2nd ed. Davos, Switzerland: AO Publishing; 2007.

Swiontkowski MF, Stovitz SD. *Manual of Orthopaedics*. 6th ed. Philadelphia, PA: Lippincott Williams & Wilkins; 2006.

Thomas Lathrop Stedman, ed. *Stedman's Concise Medical Dictionary for the Health Professions & Nursing*. 7th ed. Baltimore, MD: Lippincott Williams & Wilkins; 2011.

Thompson JC. *Netter's Concise Orthopaedic Anatomy*. 2nd ed. Philadelphia, PA: Saunders Books; 2009.

Wright JG, Swiontkowski MF, Heckman JD. Introducing levels of evidence to the journal. *J Bone Joint Surg Am*. 2003;85:1-3.

List of Appendices

Chen AF, ed.
Quick Reference Dictionary for Orthopedics (pp 198-199).

Abbreviations

AAROM: active assisted range of motion
ABC: aneurysmal bone cyst
Abd: abduction
ABG: arterial blood gas
ABI: Ankle Brachial Index
AC: acromioclavicular
ACDF: anterior cervical discectomy and fusion
ACL: anterior cruciate ligament
Add: adduction
ADL: activity of daily living
ADM: abductor digiti minimi
AF: afebrile, atrial fibrillation
AFB: acid-fast bacillus
AFO: ankle–foot orthosis
AFP: alpha-fetoprotein
AICD: automatic implanted cardiac defibrillator
AIIS: anterior inferior iliac spine
AIN: anterior interosseous nerve
AIS: adolescent idiopathic scoliosis
AKA: above-knee amputation
Alb: albumin
ALL: anterior longitudinal ligament
ALPSA: anterior labral periosteal sleeve avulsion
ALRI: anterolateral rotary instability
ALS: amyotrophic lateral sclerosis
AMA: against medical advice
AMBRI: atraumatic, multidirectional, bilateral instability
AMC: arthrogryposis multiplex congenita

Chen AF, ed.
*Quick Reference Dictionary
for Orthopedics* (pp 200-215).

ANA: antinuclear antibody
ANCOVA: analysis of covariance
ANOVA: analysis of variance
ANS: autonomic nervous system
AO: Arbeitsgemeinschaft für Osteosynthesefragen
AP: anteroposterior
A/P: assessment/plan
APB: abductor pollicis brevis
APC: anteroposterior compression
APL: abductor pollicis longus
ARDS: acute respiratory distress syndrome
AROM: active range of motion
AS: ankylosing spondylitis, aortic stenosis
ASA: anterior spinal artery, American Society of
   Anesthesiologists, aspirin
ASC: ambulatory surgery center
ASD: atrial septal defect
ASF: anterior spinal fusion
ASIF: Association for the Study of Internal Fixation
ASIS: anterior superior iliac spine
AT: athletic training
ATFL: anterotalofibular ligament
ATLS: Advanced Trauma Life Support
AVM: arteriovenous malformation
AVN: avascular necrosis

BID: twice a day
BiPAP: bilevel positive airway pressure
BKA: below-knee amputation
BM: bowel movement
BMI: body mass index
BMP: bone morphogenic protein
BP: blood pressure
BPH: benign prostatic hypertrophy
BPM: beats per minute
BR: brachioradialis
BS: blood sugar, breath sounds
BSA: body surface area
BUN: blood urea nitrogen
Bx: biopsy

Ca: calcium
CABG: coronary artery bypass graft
CAMP: cyclic adenosine monophosphate
CBC: complete blood count
CBI: closed brain injury
CC: coracoclavicular, chief complaint
CCI: Charlson Comorbidity Index
CCU: coronary care unit
CDC: Centers for Disease Control and Prevention
CDH: congenital dislocated hip
CEA: center edge angle
CF: cystic fibrosis
CHF: congestive heart failure
CHI: closed head injury
CICU: coronary intermediate care unit
CK: creatine kinase
CMC: carpometacarpal
CME: continuing medical education
CMS: Centers for Medicare and Medicaid Services
CMT: Charcot-Marie-Tooth
CN: cranial nerve
CNS: central nervous system
COPD: chronic obstructive pulmonary disease
COX: cyclooxygenase
CP: cerebral palsy, chest pain
CPAP: continuous positive airway pressure
CPK: creatinine phosphokinase
CPM: continuous passive motion
CPPD: calcium pyrophosphate dehydrate
CPR: cardiopulmonary resuscitation
CPT: current procedural terminology
CRF: chronic renal failure
CRI: chronic renal insufficiency
CRP: C reactive protein
CRPP: closed reduction and percutaneous pinning
CSF: cerebrospinal fluid
CT: computed tomography
CTL: capitotriquetral ligament
CTLSO: cervicothoracolumbosacral orthosis

CTR: carpal tunnel release
CTS: carpal tunnel syndrome
CV: cardiovascular
CVA: cerebrovascular accident, costovertebral angle
CVP: central venous pressure
Cx: culture
CXR: chest x-ray

d/c: discharge
DCMLS: dorsal column–medial lemniscus system
DCP: dynamic compression plate
DDD: degenerative disc disease
DDH: developmental dysplasia of the hip
DDx: differential diagnosis
DEXA: dual-emission x-ray absorptiometry scan
df: degrees of freedom
DFR: distal femoral replacement
DHS: dynamic hip screw
DIP: distal interphalangeal
DISH: diffuse idiopathic skeletal hyperostosis
DJD: degenerative joint disease
DKA: diabetic ketoacidosis
DM: diabetes mellitus
DMD: Duchenne muscular dystrophy
DME: durable medical equipment
DNA: deoxyribonucleic acid
DNR: do not resuscitate
DOB: date of birth
DOS: date of surgery
DP: dorsalis pedis artery
DPN: deep peroneal nerve
DRC: dorsal radiocarpal ligament
DRG: diagnosis-related groups
DRUJ: distal radioulnar joint
DT: delirium tremens
DTP: diphtheria–tetanus–pertussis
DTR: deep tendon reflex
DVT: deep vein thrombosis
Dx: diagnosis

EBM: evidence-based medicine
ECF: extracellular fluid
ECG: electrocardiogram
ECHO: echocardiogram
ECRB: extensor carpi radialis brevis
ECRL: extensor carpi radialis longus
ECU: extensor carpi ulnaris
ED: extensor digitorum, emergency department
EDB: extensor digitorum brevis
EDL: extensor digitorum longus
EDM: extensor digiti minimi
EEG: electroencephalogram
EHB: extensor hallucis brevis
EHL: extensor hallucis longus
EIP: extensor indicis proprius
EKG: electrocardiogram
EMA: epithelial membrane antigen
EMG: electromyography
ENT: ear, nose, throat
EPB: extensor pollicis brevis
EPL: extensor pollicis longus
ER: external rotation, emergency room
ESR: erythrocyte sedimentation rate
ESRD: end-stage renal disease
ETO: extended trochanteric osteotomy
EtOH: ethanol (alcohol)
EUA: exam under anesthesia
Ext: extension

FABER: flexion, abduction, external rotation
FADIR: flexion, adduction, internal rotation
FAI: femoroacetabular impingement
FAS: fetal alcohol syndrome
FB: foreign body
FBS: fasting blood sugar
FCR: flexor carpi radialis
FCU: flexor carpi ulnaris
FDB: flexor digitorum brevis
FDL: flexor digitorum longus

FDMB: flexor digiti minimi brevis
FDP: flexor digitorum profundus
FDS: flexor digitorum superficialis
FF: forward flexion
FGF: fibroblast growth factor
FGFR: fibroblast growth factor receptor
FH: family history
FHB: flexor hallucis brevis
FHL: flexor hallucis longus
FNA: fine needle aspiration
FP: family physician
FPB: flexor pollicis brevis
FPL: flexor pollicis longus
FS: frozen section
FTSG: full-thickness skin graft
FWB: full weight bearing
Fx: fracture

GABA: gamma-aminobutyric acid
GAG: glycosaminoglycan
GBS: Guillain-Barré syndrome
GCT: giant cell tumor
Gd: gadolinium
GFR: glomerular filtration rate
GH: glenohumeral, growth hormone
GI: gastrointestinal
GLAD: glenolabral articular disruption
GME: graduate medical education
GP: general practitioner
GS: Gram stain
GSW: gunshot wound
GU: genitourinary

HA: hydroxyapatite
Hct: hematocrit
HDL: high-density lipoprotein
HEP: home exercise program
Hgb: hemoglobin
HHA: home health agency

HHE: home health equipment
HHS: Harris hip score
HI: hand intrinsics
HIV: human immunodeficiency virus
HKAFO: hip–knee–ankle–foot orthosis
HMO: health maintenance organization
HMSN: hereditary motor and sensory neuropathy
HNP: herniated nucleus pulposus
HO: heterotopic ossification
H/O: history of
H&P: history and physical
HPF: high-power field
HPI: history of present illness
HR: heart rate
HSA: health systems agency
HSN: hospital satellite network
HSV: herpes simplex virus
HTN: hypertension
HV: Hemovac (Zimmer, Warsaw, Indiana)
Hx: history
Hyper: beyond or excessive
Hypo: under or lacking
Hz: hertz (cycles/second)

ICC: interclass coefficient
ICD: *International Classification of Diseases*
ICF: intracellular fluid
ICU: intensive care unit
ID: infectious disease
I&D: irrigation and debridement
IFN: interferon
Ig: immunoglobulin
IGF: insulin-like growth factor
IHSS: idiopathic hypertrophic subaortic stenosis
IJ: internal jugular
IM: intramuscular, intramedullary
INR: International Normalized Ratio
IO: intraosseous

IP: iliopsoas, interphalangeal
IR: internal rotation
IS: incentive spirometry
ISR: Insall-Salvati ratio
ITB: iliotibial band
ITT: internal tibial torsion
IU: international unit
IV: intravenous
IVC: inferior vena cava
IVDU: intravenous drug user
IVP: intravenous pressure

JP: Jackson-Pratt drain
JRA: juvenile rheumatoid arthritis

KAFO: knee–ankle–foot orthosis
KSS: Knee Society score
KUB: kidney, ureter, bladder

LAC: long arm cast
LAS: long arm splint
LBP: low-back pain
LC: lateral compression
LC-DCP: low-contact dynamic compression plate
LCFN: lateral femoral cutaneous nerve
LCH: Langerhans cell histiocytosis
LCL: lateral collateral ligament
LCP: Legg-Calvé-Perthes disease
LD: lethal dose, learning disability
LDH: lactic dehydrogenase
LDL: low-density lipoprotein
LE: lower extremity, lupus erythematosus
LH: long head
LHD: left-hand dominant
LLC: long leg cast
LLD: leg length discrepancy
LLE: left lower extremity
LLL: left lower lobe

LLQ: left lower quadrant (of abdomen)
LLS: long leg splint
LLWC: long leg walking cast
LMN: lower motor neuron
LOA: leave of absence
LOC: loss of consciousness
LOS: length of stay
LP: lumbar puncture
LS: lumbosacral
LSTV: lumbosacral transitional vertebrae
LUE: left upper extremity
LUL: left upper lobe
LVH: left ventricular hypertrophy

MAP: mean arterial pressure
MC: metacarpal, musculocutaneous
MCA: motorcycle accident
MCH: mean corpuscular hemoglobin
MCHC: mean corpuscular hemoglobin concentration
MCL: medial collateral ligament
MCP: metacarpophalangeal
MCV: mean corpuscular volume
MD: muscular dystrophy, medical doctor
MDI: multidirectional instability
MDR: multi-drug resistant
MED: multiple epiphyseal dysplasia
MEP: motor-evoked potentials
MFH: malignant fibrous histiocytoma
Mg: magnesium
MG: myesthenia gravis
MHC: myosin heavy chain
MHE: multiple hereditary exostoses
MI: myocardial infarction
MIS: minimally invasive surgery
MLD: metachromatic leukodystrophy
MM: mucous membrane, multiple myeloma
MMSE: Mini-Mental State Exam
MOM: milk of magnesia
MP: metacarpophalangeal

MPFL: medial patellofemoral ligament
MPS: mucopolysaccharidosis
MRI: magnetic resonance imaging
MRSA: methicillin-resistant *Staphylococcus aureus*
MS: mitral stenosis, multiple sclerosis
MSSA: methicillin-sensitive *Staphylococcus aureus*
MT: metatarsal
MTP: metatarsophalangeal
MUA: manipulation under anesthesia
MVA: motor vehicle accident

Na: sodium
N/A: not applicable, not available
NAD: no acute distress
NCS: nerve conduction study
NCV: nerve conduction velocity
NF: neurofibromatosis
NG: nasogastric
NICU: neonatal intensive care unit
NK: natural killer cell
NKA: no known allergy
NKDA: no known drug allergy
NP: nucleus pulposus, nurse practitioner
NPO: nothing per os (nothing by mouth)
NSAID: nonsteroidal anti-inflammatory drug
NSR: normal sinus rhythm
N/T: numbness/tingling
N/V: nausea/vomiting
NVI: neurovascularly intact
NWB: non-weight bearing

O: objective
OA: osteoarthritis
OATS: Osteochondral Autograft Transfer System
OCD: osteochondral defect
OD: overdose
ODM: opponens digiti minimi
OOB: out of bed
OPLL: ossified posterior longitudinal ligament

OR: operating room
ORIF: open reduction and internal fixation
OT: occupational therapy

P: phosphorus
PA: posteroanterior, physician assistant
PAD: peripheral arterial disease, palmar adduct
PASTA: partial articular-sided tendon avulsion
PB: palmaris brevis
PCA: patient-controlled anesthesia, posterior cerebral artery
PCL: posterior cruciate ligament
PCP: primary care physician
PDD: pervasive developmental disorder
PDR: *Physicians' Desk Reference*
PE: physical exam, pulmonary embolus, polyethylene
PEEP: positive end expiratory pressure
PERLA: pupils equal and react to light and accommodation
PET: positron emission tomography
PFR: proximal femoral replacement
PFT: pulmonary function test
PI: present illness, primary investigator
PICC: peripherally inserted central catheter
PICU: pediatric intensive care unit
PID: pelvic inflammatory disease
PIIS: posterior inferior iliac spine
PILF: posterior lumbar interbody fusion
PIN: posterior interosseous nerve
PIP: proximal interphalangeal
PKU: phenylketonuria
PL: palmaris longus
PLC: posterolateral corner
PLL: posterior longitudinal ligament
PLRI: posterolateral rotary instability
PMH: past medical history
PMMA: polymethylmethacrylate
PMRI: posteromedial rotary instability
PNA: pneumonia
PNS: peripheral nervous system

PO: per os (by mouth), postoperative
PP: percutaneous pinning
PPD: purified protein derivative
PPO: preferred provider organization
PQ: pronator quadratus
PRAFO: pressure relief ankle–foot orthosis
PRBC: packed red blood cells
PRC: proximal row carpectomy
PRE: progressive resistance exercise
PRN: pro re nata (as needed)
PROM: passive range of motion
PSF: posterior spinal fusion
PSH: past surgical history
PSIS: posterior superior iliac spine
PT: physical therapy, posterior tibialis artery, pronator teres, prothrombin, patient
PTCA: percutaneous transluminal coronary angioplasty
PTH: parathyroid hormone
PTSD: posttraumatic stress disorder
PTT: partial thromboplastin time
PTX: pneumothorax
PUS: pleomorphic undifferentiated sarcoma
PVD: peripheral vascular disease
PVNS: pigmented villonodular synovitis
PWB: partial weight bearing

Q: every
QA: quality assurance
QALY: quality-adjusted life years
QD: quaque die (once a day)
QHS: quaque hora somni (every night at bedtime)
QID: quater in die (4 times a day)
QRD: *Quick Reference Dictionary*

RA: rheumatoid arthritis
RAD: radiation absorbed dose
RANK: receptor activator of nuclear factor $\kappa\beta$
RANK-L: receptor activator of nuclear factor $\kappa\beta$ ligand
RAS: reticular activating system

RBC: red blood cell
RC: rotator cuff
RCR: rotator cuff repair
RCT: randomized controlled trial, rotator cuff tear
REM: rapid eye movement
RF: rheumatoid factor, renal failure, rheumatic fever
RHD: right-hand dominant
RIA: reamer–irrigator–aspirator
RICE: rest, ice, compress, and elevate
RLE: right lower extremity
RLL: right lower lobe
RLQ: right lower quadrant (abdomen)
RNA: ribonucleic acid
R/O: rule out
ROM: range of motion
ROS: review of systems
RPM: revolutions per minute
RSD: reflex sympathetic dystrophy
RSR: regular sinus rhythm
RUE: right upper extremity
RUL: right upper lobe
RVA: rib vertebral angle
RVH: right ventricular hypertrophy
Rx: prescription

S: subjective
SAC: short arm cast
SAD: seasonal affective disorder
SAS: short arm splint
SB: spina bifida
SBE: subacute bacterial endocarditis
SC: sternoclavicular
SCFE: slipped capital femoral epiphysis
SCI: spinal cord injury
SCM: sternocleidomastoid
SD: standard deviation
SEM: standard error of the mean
SFA: superficial femoral artery

SH: social history, short head
SI: sacroiliac
SICU: surgical intensive care unit
SIDS: sudden infant death syndrome
SILT: sensation intact to light touch
SL: scapholunate, sublingual
SLAC: scapholunate advanced collapse
SLAP: superior labrum anterior and posterior
SLC: short leg cast
SLE: systemic lupus erythematosus
SLR: straight leg raise
SLS: short leg splint
SNF: skilled nursing facility
SOB: shortness of breath
SOL: space occupying lesion
S/P: status post
SPN: superficial peroneal nerve
SQ: subcutaneous
SS: spinal stenosis
SSEP: somatosensory-evoked potential
ST: spinothalamic
STD: sexually transmitted disease
STSG: split-thickness skin graft
STT: scaphotrapeziotrapezoidal, spinothalamic tract
SVC: superior vena cava
SVT: superficial vein thrombosis, supraventricular tachycardia
Sx: symptom

TA: tibialis anterior
T&A: tonsils and adenoids
TAL: tendo-achilles lengthening
TB: tuberculosis
TBG: thyroxin-binding globulin
TBI: traumatic brain injury
TCL: transverse carpal ligament
Td: tetanus and diphtheria toxoid
TDWB: touch down weight bearing

TEA: total elbow arthroplasty
TENS: transcutaneous electrical nerve stimulation
TFCC: triangular fibrocartilage complex
TFL: tensor fascia lata
TGF-β: transforming growth factor β
THA: total hip arthroplasty
THR: total hip replacement, total hip revision
TIA: transient ischemic attack
TID: tie in die (3 times a day)
TJA: total joint arthroplasty
TKA: total knee arthroplasty
TKR: total knee replacement, total knee revision
TLC: tender loving care, total lung capacity
TLIF: transforaminal lumbar interbody fusion
TLSO: thoracolumbosacral orthosis
TMT: tarsometatarsal
TP: tibialis posterior
T-PA: tissue plasminogen activator
TPN: total parenteral nutrition
TSH: thyroid stimulating hormone
TT: tibial torsion
TTP: tender to palpation
TTWB: toe touch weight bearing
TUBS: traumatic, unilateral instability, and Bankart lesion
TURP: transurethral resection procedure
Tx: treatment

UA: urinalysis
UBC: unicameral bone cyst
UCBL: University of California Berkley Laboratory orthosis
UE: upper extremity
UGI: upper gastrointestinal
UMN: upper motor neuron
URI: upper respiratory infection
US: ultrasound
UTI: urinary tract infection
UV: ultraviolet

VA: veterans association
VAC: vacuum-assisted closure
VAS: Visual Analog Scale
VATER: vertebral, anus, trachea, esophagus, and renal
VISI: volar intercalated segment instability
VMO: vastus medialis oblique
VS: vital signs
VSD: ventricular septal defect
VSS: vital signs stable

WB: weight bearing
WBAT: weight bearing as tolerated
WBC: white blood cells
WDWN: well developed/well nourished
WE: wrist extension
WF: wrist flexion
WNL: within normal limits
Wt: weight

XR: x-ray

yo: year old (age)

Medical Roots Terminology

a-	negative prefix (n is added before words beginning with a vowel) (eg, ametria)
ab-	away from (eg, abducent)
abdomin-	abdomen (eg, abdominis, abdominoscopy)
ac-	*see* ad- (eg, accretion)
acet-	acid (eg, acetum vinegar, acetometer)
acid-	acid (eg, acidus sour, aciduric)
acou-	hear (eg, acouesthesia) (also spelled acu-)
acr-	extremity, peak (eg, acromegaly)
act-	drive, act (eg, reaction)
actin-	ray, radius (eg, actinogenesis)
acu-	hear (eg, osteoacusis)
ad-	toward (d changes to c, f, g, p, s, or t before words beginning with those consonants) (eg, adrenal)
aden-	gland (eg, adenoma)
adip-	fat (eg, adipocellular, adipose)
aer-	air (eg, anaerobiosis)
aesthe-	sensation (eg, aesthesioneurosis)
af-	*see* ad- (eg, afferent)
ag-	*see* ad- (eg, agglutinant)
-agogue	leading, inducing (eg, galactogogue)
-agra	catching, seizure (eg, podagra)
alb-	white (eg, albocinereous)
alg-	pain (eg, neuralgia, algesia)
all-	other, different (eg, allergy)
alve-	channel, cavity (eg, alveolar, alveus trough)
amb-	both, on both sides (eg, ambulate)

Chen AF, ed.
*Quick Reference Dictionary
for Orthopedics* (pp 216-235).
© 2012 Taylor & Francis Group

amph-	around, on both sides (eg, ampheclexis); *see also* amphi-
amphi-	both, doubly (i is dropped before words beginning with a vowel) (eg, amphicelous)
amyl-	starch (eg, amylosynthesis)
an-	*see* ana- (eg, anagogic)
ana-	up, positive (final a is dropped before words beginning with a vowel) (eg, anaphoresis)
andr-	man (eg, gynandroid)
angi-	vessel (eg, angiemphraxis)
ankyl-	crooked, looped (eg, ankylodactylia); also spelled ancyl-
ante-	before (eg, anteflexion)
anti-	against, counter (i is dropped before words beginning with a vowel or the word is hyphenated) (eg, antipyogenic, anti-inflammatory); *see also* contra-
antr-	cavern (eg, antrodynia)
ap-	*see* ad- (eg, append)
-aph-	touch (eg, dysaphia); *see also* hapt-
apo-	away from, detached, opposed (o is dropped before words beginning with a vowel) (eg, apophysis)
arachn-	spider (eg, arachnodactyly)
arch-	beginning, origin (eg, archenteron)
arter(i)-	elevator, artery (eg, arteriosclerosis, periarteritis)
arthr-	joint (eg, synarthrosis); *see also* articul-
articul-	articulus joint (eg, disarticulation); *see also* arthr-
as-	*see* ad- (eg, assimilation)
-ase	enzyme (eg, steatolase, proteolase)
at-	*see* ad- (eg, attrition)
aur-	ear (eg, aurinasal); *see also* ot-
aut-	self (eg, autechoscope)
auto-	self (eg, autoimmune)
aux-	increase (eg, enterauxe)
ax-	axis (eg, axofugal)
axon-	axis (eg, axonometer)

ba-	go, walk, stand (eg, hypnobatia)
bacill-	small staff, rod (eg, actinobacillosis); *see also* bacter-
bacter-	small staff, rod (eg, bacteriophage); *see also* bacill-
ball-	throw (eg, ballistics); *see also* bol-
bar-	weight (eg, pedobarometer)
bi-1	life (eg, aerobic)
bi-2	2, twice, double (eg, bipedal)
bil-	bile (eg, biliary)
blast-	bud, child, a growing thing in its early stages (eg, blastoma, zygotoblast)
blep-	look, *see* (eg, hemiablepsia)
blephar-	eyelid (eg, blepharoncus)
bol-	ball (eg, embolism)
brachi-	arm (eg, brachiocephalic)
brachy-	short (eg, brachycephalic)
brady-	slow (eg, bradycardia)
brom-	stench (eg, podobromidrosis)
bronch-	windpipe (eg, bronchoscopy)
bry-	be full of life (eg, embryonic)
bucc-	cheek (eg, distobuccal)
cac-	bad, evil, abnormal (eg, cacodontia, arthrocace); *see also* mal-, dys-
calc-1	stone, limestone, lime (eg, calcipexy)
calc-2	heel (eg, calcaneotibial)
calor-	heat (eg, calorimeter); *see also* therm-
capit-	head (eg, decapitate); *see also* cephal-
caps-	container (eg, encapsulation)
carbo-	coal, charcoal (eg, carbohydrate, carbonuria)
carcin-	crab, cancer (eg, carcinoma); *see also* cancr-
cardi-	heart (eg, lipocardiac)
cat-	*see* cata- (eg, cathode)
cata-	down, negative (final a is dropped before words beginning with a vowel) (eg, catabatic)
caud-	tail (eg, caudate)
cav-	hollow (eg, concave)

cec-	blind (eg, cecopexy)
-cele	tumor, hernia, cyst (eg, gastrocele)
cell-	room (eg, celliferous)
cen-	common (eg, cenesthesia)
cent-	100 (eg, centimeter, centipede)
cente-	puncture (eg, enterocentesis, amniocentesis)
centr-	central point, center (eg, neurocentral)
cephal-	relating to the head (eg, encephalitis)
cept-	take, receive (eg, receptor)
cer-	wax (eg, ceroplasty, ceromel)
cerebr-	relating to the cerebrum (eg, cerebrospinal)
cervic-	neck (eg, cervicitis, cervical)
chancr-	crab, cancer (eg, chancriform)
chir-	hand (eg, chiromegaly)
chlor-	green (eg, achloropsia)
chol-	bile (eg, hepatocholangeitis)
chondr-	cartilage (eg, chondromalacia)
chord-	string, cord (eg, perichordal)
chori-	protective fetal membrane (eg, endochorion)
chrom-	color (eg, polychromatic)
chron-	time (eg, synchronous)
chy-	pour (eg, ecchymosis)
-cid(e)	causing death, cut, kill (eg, infanticide, germicidal)
cili-	eyelid (eg, superciliary); *see also* blephar-
cine-	move (eg, autocinesis)
-cipient	take, receive (eg, incipient)
circum-	around (eg, circumferential); *see also* peri-
-cis-	cut, kill (eg, excision)
clas-	break (eg, osteoclast, cranioclast)
clin-	bend, incline, make lie down (eg, clinometer)
clus-	shut (eg, malocclusion)
co-	*see* con- (eg, cohesion)
cocc-	seed, pill (eg, gonococcus)
coel-	hollow (eg, coelenteron); also spelled cel-
col-1	pertaining to the lower intestine (eg, colic)
col-2	*see* con- (eg, collapse)
colon-	lower intestine (eg, colonic)
colp-	hollow, vagina (eg, endocolpitis)
com-	*see* con- (eg, commasculation)

con-	with, together (becomes co- before vowels or h; col- before l; com- before b, m, or p; cor- before r) (eg, contraction)
contra-	against, counter (eg, contraindication); *see also* anti-
copr-	dung (eg, coproma); *see also* sterco-
cor-1	doll, little image, pupil (eg, isocoria)
cor-2	*see* con- (eg, corrugator)
corpor-	body (eg, intracorporal); *see also* somat-
cortic-	bark, rind (eg, corticosterone)
cost-	rib (eg, intercostal); *see also* pleur-
crani-	skull, cranium (eg, pericranium)
creat-	meat, flesh (eg, creatorrhea)
-crescent	grow (eg, excrescent)
cret-1	grow (eg, accretion)
cret-2	distinguish, separate off (eg, discrete)
crin-	distinguish, separate off (eg, endocrinology)
crur-	shin, leg (eg, brachiocrural)
cry-	cold (eg, cryesthesia)
crypt-	hide, conceal (eg, cryptorchism)
cult-	tend, cultivate (eg, culture)
cune-	wedge (eg, sphencuneiform)
cut-	skin (eg, subcutaneous); *see also* derm(at)-
cyan-	blue (eg, anthocyanin)
cycl-	circle, cycle (eg, cyclophoria)
cyst-	bag, bladder (eg, nephrocystitis); *see also* vesic-
cyt-	cell (eg, plasmocytoma); *see also* cell-
dacry-	tear (eg, dacryocyst)
dactyl-	finger, toe, digit (eg, hexadactylism)
de-	down from (eg, decomposition)
dec-1	10, indicates multiple in metric system (eg, decagram)
dec-2	10, indicates fraction in metric system (eg, decimeter)
deci-	10th (eg, decibel)
demi-	half (eg, demipenniform)
dendr-	tree (eg, neurodendrite)
dent-	tooth (eg, interdental); *see also* odont-

derm-	skin (eg, endoderm, dermatitis); *see also* cut-
desm-	band, ligament (eg, syndesmopexy)
dextr-	handedness (eg, ambidextrous)
di-1	2 (eg, dimorphic); see also bi-2
di-2	*see* dia- (eg, diuresis)
di-3	*see* dis- (eg, divergent)
dia-	through, apart, between, asunder (a is dropped before words beginning with a vowel) (eg, diagnosis)
didym-	twin, gemini (eg, epididymal)
digit-	finger, toe (eg, digital); *see also* dactyl-
diplo-	double (eg, diplomyelia)
dis-	apart, away from, negative, absence of (s may be dropped before a word beginning with a consonant) (eg, dislocation)
disc-	disk (eg, discoplacenta)
dors-	back (eg, ventrodorsal)
drom-	course (eg, hemodromometer)
-ducent	lead, conduct (eg, adducent)
duct-	lead, conduct (eg, oviduct)
dur-	hard, sclera (eg, induration)
dynam(i)-	power (eg, dynamoneure, neurodynamic)
-dynia	pain (eg, coxodynia)
dys-	bad, improper, malfunction, difficult (eg, dystrophic)
e-	out from (eg, emission)
ec-	out of, on the outside (eg, eccentric)
-ech-	have, hold, be (eg, synechotomy)
ect-	outside (eg, ectoplasm); *see also* extra-
-ectomy	a cutting out (eg, mastectomy)
ede-	swell (eg, edematous)
ef-	out of (eg, efflorescent)
-elc-	sore, ulcer (eg, enterelcosis); *see also* helc-
electr-	amber (eg, electrotherapy)
em-	in, on (eg, embolism, empathy, emphlysis); *see also* en-
-em-	blood (eg, anemia); *see also* hem(at)-
-emesis	vomiting (eg, nemesis)

-emia	blood (eg, bacteremia)
en-	in, on, into (n changes to m before b, p, or ph) (eg, encelitis)
end-	inside (eg, endangium); *see also* intra-
endo-	within (eg, endocardium)
enter-	intestine (eg, dysentery)
epi-	upon, after, in addition (i is dropped before words beginning with a vowel) (eg, epiglottis, epaxial)
erg-	work, deed (eg, energy)
erythr-	red, rubor (eg, erythrochromia)
eso-	inside (eg, esophylactic); *see also* intra-, endo-
esthe-	perceive, feel, sensation (eg, anesthesia)
eu-	good, normal, well (eg, eupepsia, eugeric)
ex-	out of (eg, excretion)
exo-	outside (eg, exopathic); *see also* extra-
extra-	outside of, beyond (eg, extracellular)
faci-	face (eg, brachiofaciolingual)
-facient	make (eg, calefacient)
-fact-	make (eg, artifact)
fasci-	band (eg, fascia)
febr-	fever (eg, febrile, febricide)
-fect-	make (eg, defective)
-ferent	bear, carry (eg, efferent, afferent)
ferr-	iron (eg, ferroprotein)
fibr-	fiber (eg, chondrofibroma)
fil-	thread (eg, filament, filiform)
fiss-	split (eg, fissure)
flagell-	whip (eg, flagellation)
flav-	yellow (eg, riboflavin)
-flect-	bend, divert (eg, deflection)
-flex-	bend, divert (eg, reflexometer, flexion)
flu-	flow (eg, fluid)
flux-	flow (eg, affluxion)
for-	door, opening (eg, foramen, perforated)
fore-	before, in front of (eg, forefront)
-form	shape, form (eg, ossiform, cuniform)
fract-	break (eg, fracture, refractive)

front-	forehead, front (eg, nasofrontal)
-fug(e)	to drive away, flee, avoid (eg, vermifuge, centrifugal)
funct-	perform, serve, function (eg, functional, malfunction)
fund-	pour (eg, infundibulum)
fus-	pour (eg, diffusible)
galact-	milk (eg, dysgalactia)
gam-	marriage, reproductive union (eg, agamont)
gangli-	swelling, plexus (eg, neurogangliitis)
gastro-	stomach, belly (eg, gastrostomy)
gelat-	freeze, congeal (eg, gelatin)
gemin-	twin, double (eg, quadrigeminal)
gen-	become, be produced, originate, formation (eg, genesis, cytogenic, gene)
germ-	bud, a growing thing in its early stages (eg, germinal, ovigerm)
gest-	bear, carry (eg, congestion)
gland-	acorn (eg, intraglandular)
-glia	glue (eg, neuroglia)
gloss-	relating to the tongue (eg, lingutrichoglossia)
glott-	tongue, language (eg, glottic)
gluc-	sweet (eg, glucose)
glutin-	glue (eg, agglutination)
glyc(y)-	sweet (eg, glycemia, glycyrrhiza)
gnath-	jaw (eg, orthognathous)
gno-	know, discern (eg, diagnosis)
gon-	produce, formulate (eg, gonad, amphigony)
grad-	walk, take steps (eg, retrograde)
-gram	scratch, write, record (eg, cardiogram)
gran-	grain, particle (eg, lipogranuloma, granulation)
graph-	scratch, write, record (eg, histography)
grav-	heavy (eg, multigravida)
gyn(ec)-	woman, wife (eg, androgyny, gynecologic)
gyr-	ring, circle (eg, gyrospasm)
hapt-	touch (eg, haptometer)
hect-	100, indicates multiple in metric system (eg, hectometer)

helc-	sore, ulcer (eg, helcosis)
hem(at)-	blood (eg, hematocyturia, hemangioma)
hemi-	half (eg, hemiageusia); *see also* semi-
hen-	one (eg, henogenesis)
hepat-	liver (eg, gastrohepatic)
hept(a)-	7 (eg, heptatomic, heptavalent)
hered-	heir (eg, heredity)
hetero-	other, indicating dissimilarity (eg, heterogeneous)
hex-1	6, *see also* sex- (eg, hexagram)
hex-2	have, hold, be (eg, cachexy)
hexa-	6, *see also* sex- (eg, hexachromic)
hidr-	sweat (eg, hyperhidrosis)
hist-	web, tissue (eg, histodialysis)
hod-	road, path (eg, hodoneuromere)
holo-	all (eg, hologenesis)
homo-	common, same (eg, homomorphic)
horm-	impetus, impulse (eg, hormone)
hydat-	water (eg, hydatism)
hydr-	pertaining to water (eg, achlorhydria)
hyp-	under (eg, hypaxial, hypodermic)
hyper-	over, above, beyond, extreme (eg, hypertrophy)
hypn-	sleep (eg, hypnotic)
hypo-	under, below (o is dropped before words beginning with a vowel) (eg, hypometabolism)
hyster-	womb (eg, hysterectomy)
-iasis	condition, pathological state (eg, hemiathriasis); *see also* -osis
iatr-	specialty in medicine (eg, pediatrics)
idio-	peculiar, separate, distinct (eg, idiosyncrasy)
il-1	negative prefix (eg, illegible)
il-2	in, on (eg, illinition)
ile-	pertaining to the ileum (ile- is commonly used to refer to the portion of the intestines known as the ileum) (eg, ileostomy)
ili-	lower abdomen, intestines (ili- is commonly used to refer to the flaring part of the hip bone known as the ilium) (eg, iliosacral)
im-1	in, on (eg, immersion)

im-2	negative prefix (eg, imperfection)
in-1	fiber (eg, inosteatoma)
in-2	in, on (n changes to l, m, or r before words beginning with those consonants) (eg, insertion)
in-3	negative prefix (eg, invalid)
infra-	beneath (eg, infraorbital)
insul-	island (eg, insulin)
inter-	among, between (eg, intercarpal)
intra-	inside (eg, intravenous)
ir-1	in, on (eg, irradiation)
ir-2	negative prefix (eg, irreducible)
irid-	rainbow, colored circle (eg, keratoiridocyclitis)
is-	equal (eg, isotope)
ischi-	hip, haunch (eg, ischiopubic)
-ism	condition, theory (eg, hemiballism, agism)
iso-	equal (eg, isotonic)
-itis	inflammation (eg, neuritis)
-ize	to treat by special method (eg, specialize)
jact-	throw (eg, jactitation)
ject-	throw (eg, injection)
jejun-	hungry, not partaking of food (eg, gastrojejunostomy)
jug-	yoke (eg, conjugation)
junct-	yoke, join (eg, conjunctiva)
juxta-	near (eg, juxtaposed)
kary-	nut, kernel, nucleus (eg, megakaryocyte)
kerat-	horn (eg, keratolysis, keratin)
kil-	1000, indicates multiple in metric system (eg, kilogram)
kine-	move (eg, kinematics)
-kinesis	movement (eg, orthokinesis)
labi-	lip (eg, gingivolabial)
lact-	milk (eg, glucolactone, lactose)
lal-	talk, babble (eg, glossolalia)
lapar-	flank, loin, abdomen (eg, laparotomy)
laryng-	windpipe (eg, laryngendoscope)

lat-	bear, carry (eg, translation)
later-	side (eg, bentrolateral)
lent-	lentil (eg, lenticonus)
lep-	take, seize (eg, cataleptic, epileptic)
lepto-	small, soft (eg, leptotene)
leuk-	white (eg, leukocyte); also spelled leuc-
lien-	spleen (eg, lienocele)
lig-	tie, bind (eg, ligate)
lingu-	tongue (eg, sublingual)
lip-	fat (eg, glycolipid)
lith-	stone (eg, nephrolithotomy)
loc-	place (eg, locomotion)
log-	speak, give an account (eg, logorrhea, embryology)
lumb-	loin (eg, dorsolumbar)
lute-	yellow (eg, xanthluteoma)
ly-	loose, dissolve (eg, keratolysis)
-lysis	setting free, disintegration (eg, glycolysis)
lymph-	water (eg, hydrolymphadenosis)
macro-	long, large (eg, macromyoblast)
mal-	bad, abnormal (eg, malfunction)
malac-	soft (eg, osteomalacia)
mamm-	breast (eg, mammogram, mammary)
man-	hand (eg, maniphalanx, manipulation)
mani-	mental aberration (eg, kleptomania)
mast-	breast (eg, mastectomy, hypermastia)
medi-	middle (eg, medial, medifrontal)
mega-	great, large, indicates multiple (1,000,000) in metric system (eg, megacolon, megadyne)
megal-	great, large (eg, cardiomegaly, acromegaly)
mel-	limb, member (eg, symmelia)
melan-	black (eg, melanoma, melanin)
men-	month (eg, menopause, dysmenorrhea)
mening-	membrane (eg, encephalomeningitis)
ment-	mind (eg, dementia)
mer-	part (eg, polymeric)
mes-	middle (eg, mesoderm)
met-	after, beyond, accompanying (eg, metallurgy)

meta-	after, beyond, accompanying (a is dropped before words beginning with a vowel) (eg, metacarpal, metatarsal)
metr-1	measure (eg, stereometry)
metr-2	womb (eg, endometritis)
micr-	small (eg, photomicrograph)
mill-	1000, indicates fraction in metric system (eg, milligram, millipede)
mio-	smaller, less (eg, mionectic)
miss-	send (eg, intromission)
-mittent	send (eg, intermittent)
mne-	remember (eg, pseudoamnesia)
mon-	only, sole, single (eg, monoplegia)
morph-	form, shape (eg, morphonuclear)
mot-	move (eg, vasomotor, locomotion)
multi-	many (eg, multiple)
my-	muscle (eg, myopathy)
-myces	fungus (eg, myelomyces)
myc(et)-	fungus (eg, ascomycetes, streptomycin)
myel-	marrow (eg, poliomyelitis)
myx-	mucus (eg, myxedema)
narc-	numbness (eg, toponarcosis, narcolepsy)
nas-	nose (eg, nasal)
ne-	new, young (eg, neocyte, neonate)
necr-	corpse, dead (eg, necrocytosis, necrosis)
nephr-	kidney (eg, nephron, nephric)
neur-	nerve (eg, neurology, esthesioneure)
nod-	knot (eg, nodosity)
nom-	deal out, distribute, law, custom (eg, nominal, taxonomy)
non-	nine, no (eg, nonacosane)
nos-	disease (eg, nosology)
nucle-	nut, kernel (eg, nucleus, nucleide)
nutri-	nourish (eg, malnutrition)
ob-	against, toward (b changes to c before words beginning with that consonant) (eg, obtuse)
oc-	*see* ob-, occlude

ocul-	eye (eg, oculomotor)
-od-	road, path (eg, periodic)
-ode-1	road, path (eg, cathode)
-ode-2	form (eg, nematode)
odont-	tooth (eg, orthodontia)
-odyn-	pain, distress (eg, gastrodynia)
-oid	form (eg, hyoid)
-ol	oil (eg, cholesterol)
-old	form, shape, resemblance (eg, scaffold)
ole-	oil (eg, oleoresin)
olig-	few, small (eg, oligospermia)
-oma	tumor (eg, blastoma)
omo-	shoulder (eg, omosternum)
omphal-	navel (eg, periomphalic)
onc-	bulk, mass (eg, oncology, hematoncometry)
onych-	claw, nail (eg, anonychia)
oo-	egg, ovum (eg, perioothecitis)
oophor-	pertaining to the ovary (eg, oophorectomy)
ophthalm-	eye (eg, ophthalmic)
or-	mouth (eg, intraoral)
orb-	circle (eg, suborbital)
orchi-	testicle (eg, orchiopathy)
organ-	implement, instrument (eg, organoleptic)
orth-	straight, right, normal (eg, orthopedics)
-osis	condition, disease (eg, osteoporosis)
oss-	bone (eg, osseous, ossiphone)
ost(e)-	bone (eg, enostosis, osteonecrosis)
ot-	ear (eg, parotid); *see also* aur-
-otomy	cutting (eg, osteotomy)
ov-	egg (eg, synovia)
oxy-	sharp, acid (eg, oxycephalic)
pachy(n)-	thicken (eg, pachyderma, myopachynsis)
pag-	fix, make fast (eg, thoracopagus)
pan-	entire, all (eg, pancytosis, pandemic)
par-1	bear, give birth to (eg, primiparous)
par-2	*see* para- (eg, parepigastric)
para-	beside, beyond, alongside of (final a is dropped before words beginning with a vowel) (eg, paramastoid)

part-	bear, give birth to (eg, parturition)
path-	that which one undergoes, sickness, disease (eg, pathology, psychopathic)
pec-	fix, make fast (eg, sympectothiene); *see also* pex-
ped-	child (eg, pediatric, orthopedic)
pell-	skin, hide (eg, pellagra)
-pellent	drive (eg, repellent)
pen-	need, lack (eg, erythrocytopenia)
pend-	hang down (eg, appendix)
pent(a)-	5 (eg, pentose, pentaploid)
peps-	digest (eg, bradypepsia)
pept-	digest (eg, dyspeptic)
per-	through, excessive (eg, pernasal)
peri-	around (eg, periphery)
pet-	seek, tend toward (eg, centripetal)
pex-	fix, make fast (eg, hepatopexy)
pha-	say, speak (eg, dysphasia)
phac-	lentil, lens (eg, phacosclerosis); also spelled phak-
phag-	eat (eg, lipphagic)
phak-	lentil, lens (eg, phakitis)
phan-	show, be seen (eg, diaphanoscopy)
pharmac-	drug (eg, pharmacology)
pharyng-	throat (eg, glossopharyngeal)
phen-	show, be seen (eg, phosphene)
pher-	bear, support (eg, periphery)
phil-	like, have affinity for (eg, eosinophilia, philosophy)
phleb-	vein (eg, periphlebitis, phlebotomy)
phleg-	burn, inflame (eg, adenophlegmon)
phlog-	burn, inflame (eg, antiphlogistic)
phob-	fear, dread (eg, claustrophobia)
phon-	sound (eg, echophony)
phor-	bear, support (eg, exophoria)
phos-	light (eg, phosphorus)
phot-	light (eg, photerythrous)
phrag-	fence, wall off, stop up (eg, diaphragm)
phrax-	fence, wall off, stop up (eg, emphraxis)
phren-	mind, midriff (eg, metaphrenia, metaphrenon)
phthi-	decay, waste away (eg, ophthalmophthisis)

phy-	beget, bring forth, produce, be by nature (eg, nosophyte, physical)
phyl-	tribe, kind (eg, phylogeny)
phylac-	guard (eg, prophylactic)
-phylaxis	protection (eg, prophylaxis)
-phyll	leaf (eg, xanthophyll)
phys(a)-	blow, inflate (eg, physocele, physalis)
physe-	blow, inflate (eg, emphysema)
pil-	hair (eg, epilation)
pituit-	phlegm (eg, pituitous)
placent-	cake (eg, extraplacental)
plas-	mold, shape (eg, cineplasty, plastazode)
platy-	broad, flat (eg, platyrrhine)
pleg-	strike (eg, diplegia, paraplegia)
plet-	fill (eg, depletion)
pleur-	rib, side (eg, peripleural)
plex-	strike (eg, apoplexy)
plic-	fold (eg, complication)
plur-	more (eg, plural)
pne-	breathing (eg, traumatopnea)
pneum(at)-	breath, air (eg, pneumodynamics, pneumato-thorax)
pneumo(n)-	lung (eg, pneumocentesis, pneumonotomy)
pod-	foot (eg, podiatry)
poie-	make, produce (eg, sarcopoietic)
pol-	axis of a sphere (eg, peripolar)
poly-	much, many (eg, polyspermia)
pont-	bridge (eg, pontocerebellar)
por-1	passage (eg, myelopore)
por-2	callus (eg, porocele)
posit-	put, place (eg, deposit, repositor)
post-	after, behind in time or place (eg, postnatal, postural)
pre-	before in time or place (eg, prenatal, prevesical)
press-	press (eg, pressure, pressoreceptive)
pro-	before in time or place (eg, progamous, prolapse)
proct-	anus (eg, ecteroproctia)
prosop-	face (eg, prosopus)

proto-	first (eg, prototype)
pseud-	false (eg, pseudoparaplegia)
psych-	soul, mind (eg, psychosomatic)
pto-	fall (eg, nephroptosis)
pub-	adult (eg, puberty, ischiopubic)
puber-	adult (eg, puberty)
pulmo(n)-	lung (eg, cardiopulmonary, pulmolith)
puls-	drive (eg, propulsion)
punct-	prick, pierce (eg, puncture, punctiform)
pur-	pus (eg, puration)
py-	pus (eg, nephropyosis)
pyel-	trough, basin, pelvis (eg, nephropyelitis)
pyl-	door, orifice (eg, pylephlebitis)
pyr-	fire (eg, galactopyra)
quadr-	4 (eg, quadriplegic, quadrigeminal)
quinque-	5 (eg, quinquecuspid)
rachi-	spine (eg, alorachidian)
radi-	ray (eg, irradiation)
re-	back, again (eg, retraction)
ren-	kidneys (eg, adrenal)
ret-	net (eg, retothelium)
retro-	backwards (eg, retrodeviation, retrograde)
rhag-	break, burst (eg, hemorrhagic)
rhaph-	suture, stitching (eg, gastrorrhaphy)
rhe-	flow, discharge (eg, diarrheal)
rhex-	break, burst (eg, metrorrhexis)
rhin-	nose (eg, basirhinal)
rot-	wheel (eg, rotator)
rub(r)-	red (eg, bilirubin, rubrospinal)
sacchar-	sugar (eg, saccharin)
sacro-	pertaining to the sacrum (eg, sacroiliac)
salping-	tube, trumpet (eg, salpingitis)
sanguin-	blood (eg, sanguineous)
sarc-	flesh (eg, sarcoma)
schis-	split (eg, schistorachis, rachischisis)
scler-	hard (eg, sclerosis, scleroderma)

scop-	look at, observe (eg, endoscope)
sect-	cut (eg, sectile, resection)
semi-	half (eg, semiflexion)
sens-	perceive, feel (eg, sensory)
sep-	rot, decay (eg, sepsis)
sept-1	fence, wall off, stop up (eg, septal)
sept-2	7 (eg, septan)
ser-	whey, watery substance (eg, serum, serosynovitis)
sex-	6 (eg, sexdigitate)
sial-	saliva (eg, polysialia)
sin-	hollow, fold (eg, sinobronchitis)
sit-	food (eg, parasitic)
solut-	loose, dissolve, set free (eg, dissolution)
-solvent	loose, dissolve (eg, dissolvent)
somat-	body (eg, somatic, psychosomatic)
-some	body (eg, dictyosome)
spas-	draw, pull (eg, spasm, spastic)
spectr-	appearance, what is seen (eg, spectrum, micro-spectroscope)
sperm(at)-	seed (eg, spermacrasia, spermatozoon)
spers-	scatter (eg, dispersion)
sphen-	wedge (eg, sphenoid)
spher-	ball (eg, hemisphere)
sphygm-	pulsation (eg, sphygmomanometer)
spin-	spine (eg, cerebrospinal)
spirat-	breathe (eg, inspiratory)
splanchn-	entrails, viscera (eg, neurosplanchnic)
splen-	spleen (eg, splenomegaly)
spor-	seed (eg, sporophyte, sygospore)
squam-	scale (eg, squamous, desquamation)
sta-	make stand, stop (eg, genesistasis)
stal-	send (eg, peristalsis); *see also* stol-
staphyl-	bunch of grapes, uvula (eg, staphylococcus, staphylectomy)
stear-	fat (eg, stearodermia)
steat-	fat (eg, steatopygous)
sten-	narrow, compressed (eg, stenocardia)
ster-	solid (eg, cholesterol)
sterc-	dung (eg, stercoporphyrin)

sthen-	strength (eg, asthenia)
stol-	send (eg, diastole)
stom(at)-	mouth, orifice (eg, anastomosis, stomatogastric)
strep(h)-	twist (eg, strephosymbolia, streptomycin); *see also* stroph-
strict-	draw tight, compress, cause pain (eg, constriction)
-stringent	draw tight, compress, cause pain (eg, astringent)
stroph-	twist (eg, astrophic); *see also* strep(h)-
struct-	pile up (against) (eg, obstruction)
sub-	under, below (b changes to f or p before words beginning with those consonants) (eg, sublumbar)
suf-	*see* sub- (eg, suffusion)
sup-	*see* sub- (eg, suppository)
super-	above, beyond, extreme (eg, supermobility)
sy-	*see* syn- (eg, systole)
syl-	*see* syn- (eg, syllepsiology)
sym-	*see* syn- (eg, symbiosis, symmetry, sympathetic, symphysis)
syn-	with, together (n disappears before s, changes to l before l, and changes to m before b, m, p, and ph) (eg, myosynizesis)
ta-	stretch, put under pressure (eg, ectasis)
tac-	order, arrange (eg, atactic)
tact-	touch (eg, contact)
tax-	order, arrange (eg, ataxia, taxonomy)
tect-	cover (eg, protective)
teg-	cover (eg, integument)
tel-	end (eg, telosynapsis)
tele-	at a distance (eg, teleceptor, telescope)
tempor-	time, timely or fatal spot, temple (eg, temporomalar)
ten(ont)-	tightly stretched band (eg, tenodynia, tenonitis, tenon-, tagra)
tens-	stretch (eg, extensor)
test-	pertaining to the testicle (eg, testitis)
tetra-	4 (eg, tetragenous)
the-	put, place (eg, synthesis)

thec-	repository, case (eg, thecal)
thel-	teat, nipple (eg, thelerethism)
therap-	treatment (eg, hydrotherapy)
therm-	heat (eg, diathermy)
thi-	sulfur (eg, thiogenic)
thorac-	chest (eg, thoracoplasty)
thromb-	lump, clot (eg, thrombophlebitis, thrombopenia)
thym-	spirit (eg, dysthymia)
thyr-	shield, shaped like a door (eg, thyroid)
tme-	cut (eg, axonotmesis)
toc-	childbirth (eg, dystocia)
tom-	cut (eg, appendectomy)
ton-	stretch, put under pressure (eg, tonus, peritoneum)
top-	place (eg, topesthesia)
tors-	twist (eg, extorsion)
tox-	arrow poison, poison (eg, toxemia)
trache-	windpipe (eg, tracheotomy)
trachel-	neck (eg, trachelopexy)
tract-	draw, drag (eg, protraction)
trans-	across (eg, transport)
traumat-	wound (eg, traumatic)
tri-	3 (eg, trigonad)
trich-	hair (eg, trichoid)
trip-	rub (eg, entripsis)
trop-	turn, react (eg, sitotropism)
troph-	nurture, relating to nourishment (eg, atrophy)
tuber-	swelling, node (eg, tubercle, tuberculosis)
typ-	type (eg, atypical)
typh-	for, stupor (eg, adenotyphus)
typhl-	blind (eg, typhlectasis)
uni-	one (eg, unioval)
ur-	urine (eg, polyuria)
vacc-	cow (eg, vaccine)
vagin-	sheath (eg, invaginated)
vas-	vessel (eg, vascular)
ventro-	abdomen, in front of (eg, ventrolateral, ventrose)
vers-	turn (eg, inversion)

vert-	turn (eg, diverticulum)
vesic-	bladder (eg, vesicovaginal)
vit-	life (eg, devitalize)
vuls-	pull, twitch (eg, convulsion)
xanth-	yellow, blond (eg, xanthophyll)
-yl-	substance (eg, cacodyl)
zo-	life, animal (eg, microzoaria)
zyg-	yoke, union (eg, zygote, zygodactyly)
zym-	ferment (eg, enzyme)

Anatomical Terms (Orientation and Direction)

anterior: front, ventral

anteroposterior: front to back

caudal: toward the tail (or feet)

cephalad: toward the head

cranial: relating to the head

decubitus: lying down

deep: underneath, further from the surface

distal: further from the beginning, further from the trunk

dorsal: back, posterior

horizontal: parallel to the floor, perpendicular to a vertical line

inferior: below, lower than

lateral: toward the side of the body

medial: toward the midline of the body

posterior: back, dorsal

posteroanterior: from back to front

pronation: internal rotation of the forearm so as to place the palm down

prone: with the front or ventral surface down, lying face down

proximal: closer toward the beginning, closer to the trunk

recumbent: lying down

sagittal: A vertical plane passing through the body from front to back. The midsagittal plane divides the body into left and right halves.

superficial: on top, near the surface, shallow

Chen AF, ed.
Quick Reference Dictionary for Orthopedics (pp 236-237).

superior: above

supination: external rotation of the forearm so as to place the palm up

supine: with the back or dorsal surface downward, lying face up

transverse: a horizontal plane (parallel to the ground) passing through the body

ventral: front, anterior

vertical: upright, perpendicular to horizontal

Anatomy—Muscles (Insertion, Origin, Innervation)

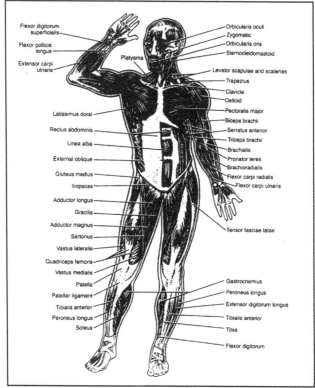

Figure 4-1. Anterior superficial muscles. (Reprinted with permission from Leonard P. *Quick and Easy Terminology*. 2nd ed. Philadelphia, PA: WB Saunders; 1995.)

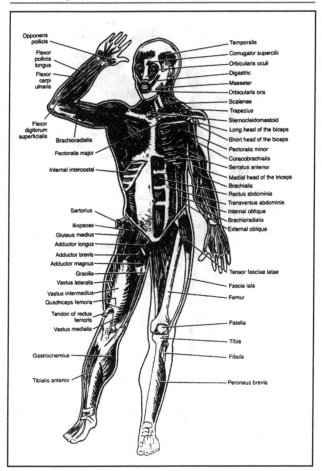

Figure 4-2. Anterior deep muscles. (Reprinted with permission from Leonard P. *Quick and Easy Terminology.* 2nd ed. Philadelphia, PA: WB Saunders; 1995.)

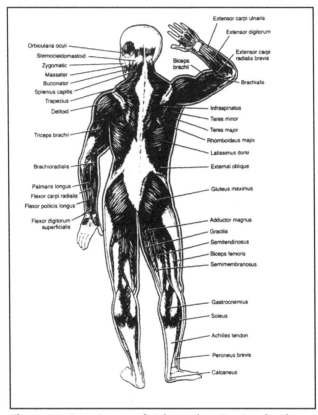

Figure 4-3. Posterior superficial muscles. (Reprinted with permission from Leonard P. *Quick and Easy Terminology*. 2nd ed. Philadelphia, PA: WB Saunders; 1995.)

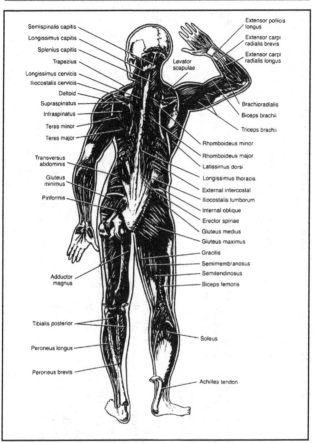

Figure 4-4. Anterior deep muscles. (Reprinted with permission from Leonard P. *Quick and Easy Terminology*. 2nd ed. Philadelphia, PA: WB Saunders; 1995.)

MUSCLES: ORIGIN/INSERTION/ACTION—INNERVATION—BLOOD SUPPLY*

Muscle	Origin	Insertion	Action	Nerve	Artery
Neck					
Sternocleido-mastoid (SCM)	Med or sternal head cranial part of ventral surface of manubrium; lat or clavicular head—sup border & ant surface of med 1/3 clavicle	Lat surface mastoid process & lat 1/2 sup nuchal line of occipital bone	↻ opp side lat ✓ same side ✓ forward	Spinal accessory n. C2 & C3 ant rami	Subclavian a.
Platysma	Fascia covering sup part of pectoralis major & deltoid	Some fibers into bone below oblique line, others into skin	Draws lip inf & post	Cervical branch of facial n.	Subclavian a. (branch)
Suprahyoid Group					
Digastricus	Post belly: mastoid notch of temporal bone; Ant belly: a depression on inner side of inf border of mandible	Post belly: hyoid bone by fibrous loop; Ant belly: same as post belly	▲ hyoid bone Post: draws backward Ant: draws forward	Post: facial n. Ant: mylohyoid n.	Lingual a.
Stylohyoideus	Post & lat surface of styloid process	Body of hyoid bone	Draws hyoid sup & post	Facial n. (branch)	Lingual a.

Note: Please refer to key on page 266.

Muscle	Origin	Insertion	Action	Nerve	Artery
Neck					
Mylohyoideus	Whole length of mylohyoid line of mandible	Body of hyoid bone	▲ hyoid & tongue	Mylohyoid n.	Lingual a.
Geniohyoideus	Inf mental spine on inner surface of symphysis menti	Ant surface of hyoid	Draws hyoid & tongue ant	1st cervical n. (through hypoglossal n.)	Lingual a.
Infrahyoid Group					
Sternohyoideus	Post surface of med end of clavicle, post sternoclavicular ligament & sup & post part of manubrium sterni	Inf border of hyoid bone	Draws hyoid inferiorly	Branch of ansa cervicalis (1st 3 cervical nerves)	Lingual a. Subclavian a.
Sternothyroideus	Dorsal surface of manubrium sterni (caudal of origin of sternohyoideus)	Oblique line on lamina of thyroid cartilage	Draws thyroid caudally	Branch of ansa cervicalis (1st 3 cervical nerves)	Subclavian a.
Thyrohyoideus	Oblique line on lamina of thyroid cartilage	Inf border of greater cornu of hyoid bone	Draws hyoid inferiorly Draws thyroid cartilage sup	1st & 2nd cervical n.	Lingual a. Subclavian a.
Omohyoideus	Cranial border of scapula (near or crossing scapular notch)	Caudal border of hyoid bone	Draws hyoid caudally	Branch of ansa cervicalis (1st 3 cervical nerves)	Subclavian a.

Neck

Muscle	Origin	Insertion	Action	Nerve	Artery
Longus Colli	Vertical: ant surface of C5, C6, C7, T1, T2 & T3; Sup: ant tubercles of transverse processes C3, C4, C5; Inf: ant surface of T2 & T3	Vertical: ant surface of C2, C3, C4; Sup: narrow tendon into tubercle on ant arch of atlas; Inf: ant tubercles of transverse processes C5 & C6	✓ neck; ↻ neck (min)	Branches of 2nd to 7th cervical n.	Subclavian a. (thyrocervical)
Longus Capitus	4 tendinous slips from ant tubercles of transverse processes C3, C4, C5 & C6	Inf surface of the basilar part of occipital bone	Head ✓	Branches from 1st, 2nd, & 3rd cervical n.	Subclavian a.
Rectus Capitus Anterior	Ant surface of lat mass of the atlas & from root of its transverse process	Inf surface of basilar part of occipital bone	Head ✓	Branch of 1st & 2nd cervical n.	Subclavian a.
Rectus Capitus Lateralis	Sup surface of transverse process of atlas	Inf surface of jugular process of occipital bone	Lat ✓ head	Branch of 1st & 2nd cervical n.	Subclavian a.
Scalenus Anterior	Ant tubercles of transverse processes of C3, C4, C5 & C6	Scalene tubercle on inner border of 1st rib & ridge on cranial surface of rib	▲ 1st rib; ✓ head; ↻ head	Branches of lower cervical n.	Subclavian a. (thyrocervical)

Muscle	Origin	Insertion	Action	Nerve	Artery
Back/Neck					
Scalenus Medius	Post tubercles of transverse processes of C2, C3, C4, C5, C6 & C7	Cranial surface of 1st rib between tubercle & subclavian groove	▲ 1st rib ↙ head ↻ head	Branches from cervical n.	Subclavian a. (thyrocervical)
Scalenus Posterior	Post tubercles of transverse processes of C5, C6 & C7	Outer surface of 2nd rib (deep to serratus anterior)	▲ 2nd rib ↙ head ↻ head	Ventral primary branches C5, C6 & C7	Subclavian a.
Back/Neck					
Serratus Posterior Superior	Caudal part of ligamentum nuchae, spinous processes C7, T1, T2 & T3; supraspinal ligament	4 digitations—cranial borders of ribs 2, 3, 4 & 5	Respiratory ▲ ribs	Ventral rami T1 to T4	Subclavian a.
Serratus Posterior Inferior	Spinous processes T11, T12, L1, L2 & L3; supraspinal ligament	4 digitations into inf borders last 4 ribs (a little beyond their angles)	Respiratory Draws ribs ◀▶ & ▼	Ventral rami T9 to T12	Subclavian a.
Splenius Capitis Cervicis	Caudal 1/2 ligamentum nuchae & spinous processes C7, T1, T2, T3 & sometimes T4	Occipital bone just inf to lat 1/3 of sup nuchal line; into mastoid process of temporal bone	↗ head&neck lat ✓ same side ↻ same side	Lat branches dorsal primary cervical n.	Subclavian a. (branches)

Muscle	Origin	Insertion	Action	Nerve	Artery
Back/Neck					
Spinalis Capitis	Usually inseparable from semispinalis capitis	Usually inseparable from semispinalis capitis	/ spine	Branch dorsal primary spinal nerves	Thoracic aorta (branch)
Semispinalis Capitis	Tips of transverse processes C7, T1, T2, T3, T4, T5, T6 & sometimes T7	Between sup & inf nuchal lines of occipital bone	/ head & neck ↻ opp side	Dorsal rami	Subclavian a. (branches)
Longissimus Capitis	Transverse processes T4 & T5 and cervicis & articular processes C4 C5, C6 & C7	Post margin of mastoid process (deep to splenius capitis & SCM)	/ head ↻ same side ✓ same side	Dorsal primary mid & lower cervical n(s).	Subclavian a. (branches)
Obliquus Capitis Inferior	Arises from apex of spinous process of axis	Inf & dorsal transverse process of atlas	↻ same side	Branch dorsal primary division suboccipital n.	Subclavian a. (branch)
Obliquus Capitis Superior	Tendinous fibers from sup surface transverse process of atlas	Occipital bone between sup & inf nuchal lines (lat to semispinalis capitis)	/ head	Branch dorsal primary division suboccipital n.	Subclavian a. (branch)
Rectus Capitis Posterior Major	Spinous process of the axis	Lat part of inf nuchal line of occipital bone and surface immediately inf	/ head ↻ same side	Branch dorsal primary division suboccipital n.	Subclavian a. (branch)

Back

Muscle	Origin	Insertion	Action	Nerve	Artery
Rectus Capitis Posterior Minor	Tendon from tubercle on post arch of atlas	Med part of the inf nuchal line of occipital bone & surface between it & foramen magnum	/ head	Branch dorsal primary division suboccipital n.	Subclavian a. (branch)
Longissimus Cervicis	Long thin tendons from apex transverse processes upper 4 or 5 thoracic vertebrae	Post tubercles of transverse processes of C2 to C6	/ spine lat ✓ ▼ ribs	Dorsal primary branch spinal n.	Thoracic aorta (branches)
Iliocostalis Cervicis	Angles of the 3rd, 4th, 5th & 6th ribs	Post tubercles of transverse processes of C4, C5 & C6	/ spine lat ✓ ▼ ribs	Dorsal primary branch spinal n.	Thoracic aorta (branches)
Spinalis Cervicis	Caudal part of ligamentum nuchae, spinous process C7; sometimes T1 & T2	Spinous processes of axis; sometimes spinous process C1 & C2	/ spine	Dorsal primary branch spinal n.	Thoracic aorta (branch)
Semispinalis Cervicis	Transverse processes of 1st 5 or 6 thoracic vertebrae	Cervical spinous processes from axis to C5	/ spine ↻ opp side	Dorsal primary branch spinal n.	Thoracic aorta (branch)

Muscle	Origin	Insertion	Action	Nerve	Artery
Back					
Longissimus Thoracis	Arising from erector spinae & post surfaces transverse & accessory processes of lumbar vertebrae & ant layer lumbocostal aponeurosis	Transverse processes of all thoracic vertebrae and lower 9 or 10 ribs between tubercles and angles	/ spine lat ✓ ▼ ribs	Dorsal primary branch spinal n.	Thoracic aorta (branch)
Iliocostalis Thoracis	Flattened tendons from upper borders of angles of lower 6 ribs (med to iliocostalis lumborum)	Cranial borders of angles of 1st 6 ribs and into dorsum of transverse process C7	/ spine lat ✓ ▼ ribs	Dorsal primary branch spinal n.	Thoracic aorta (branch)
Spinalis Thoracis	Med continuation of sacrospinalis. Arises from spinous processes of T11, T12, L1 & L2	Spinous processes of upper thoracic vertebrae	/ spine	Dorsal primary branch spinal n.	Thoracic aorta (branch)
Semispinalis Thoracis	Transverse processes of T6 to T10	Spinous processes of C6, C7, T1, T2, T3 & T4	/ spine ↻ opp side	Dorsal primary branch spinal n.	Thoracic aorta (branch)
Iliocostalis Lumborum	Flattened tendons from upper portion of erector	Inf borders of angles of last 6 or 7 ribs	/ spine lat ✓ ▼ ribs	Dorsal primary branch spinal n.	Thoracic aorta (branch)

Back

Muscle	Origin	Insertion	Action	Nerve	Artery
Sacrospinalis (Erector Spinae)	Arises from broad tendon attached to mid crest of sacrum; spinous processes T11 to T12 & lumbar vertebrae; supraspinal ligament to lip of iliac crests & lat crest of sacrum	Splits into longissimus, iliocostalis, spinalis, & semispinalis muscles (see respective muscles)	↗ spine ↻ spine ▼ ribs lat ✓	Spinal n.	Thoracic aorta
Multifidus	Spinous processes of each vertebra from sacrum to axis; arises from back of sacrum from aponeurosis of sacrospinalis, from med surface of post sup iliac spine & post sacroiliac ligaments	Each ascends obliquely crossing over 2 to 4 vertebrae and inserted into spinous process of vertebra from last lumbar to axis	↗ spine ↻ opp side	Branches of dorsal primary spinal n.	Thoracic aorta
Rotatores	Transverse process of one vertebra & insert at base of spinous process of vertebra above from the sacrum to the axis	*Rotatores longi* cross one vertebra in their oblique course. *Rotatores breves* insert in next succeeding vertebra & run horizontal	↗ spine ↻ opp side	Branches of dorsal primary spinal n.	Thoracic aorta

Muscle	Origin	Insertion	Action	Nerve	Artery
Shoulder Girdle					
Quadratus Lumborum	Sup borders of the transverse processes L2 to L5	Inf border of last rib & transverse process L1 to L4	▼ last rib lat ✓	12th thoracic n. 1st lumbar n.	Iliac circumflex
Shoulder Girdle					
Trapezius	Ext occipital protuberance; med 1/3 sup nuchal line; spinous process C7, T1 to T12	Post border of lat 3rd clavicle; med margin acromion; spine of the scapula	▲ &/shoulder Abd same side ↻ opp side Retraction ▲ ↻ glen fossa ▲ glen fossa	Spinal accessory n. C3 & C4 spinal n.	Suprascapular a.
Levator Scapulae	Transverse processes C1 to C4	Med border scapula between sup angle & spine	Elevation Protraction / cervical spine Abd same side ↻ same side	Dorsal scapular n. C3 & C4 spinal n.	Superficial cervical a. Transverse cervical a.
Romboideus Minor	Spinous process of C7 & T1	Med border scapula at level of the spine	Elevation Retraction ▼ ↻ glen fossa	Dorsal scapular n.	Descending scapular a.
Romboideus Major	Spinous process of T2 to T5	Med border scapula between spine & inf angle	Elevation Retraction ▼ ↻ glen fossa	Dorsal scapular n.	Descending scapular a.

Shoulder Girdle

Muscle	Origin	Insertion	Action	Nerve	Artery
Latissimus Dorsi	Lumbar aponeurosis; spinous processes of T6 to T12, L1 to L5 & sacral vertebrae	Distal part of intertubercular groove of humerus	/ shoulder Abd shoulder Med ↻ Elevation Retraction	Thoracodorsal n. C6-C8 spinal n.	Subscapular a.
Pectoralis Major	Ant surface sternal 1/2 clavicle; ventral surface sternum; aponeurosis of obliquus externus abdominis	Crest of greater tubercle of humerus	✓ shoulder Add shoulder Med ↻ Protract; ▲▼	Med & lat pectoral n. C5 to C8 spinal nerves 1st thoracic n.	Thoracoacromial a.
Pectoralis Minor	Ext surfaces of ribs 3, 4 & 5 near their cartilages	Caracoid process of scapula	Protraction Depression ▼ ↻ glen fossa	Med pectoral n.	Thoracoacromial a.
Subclavius	1st rib & its cartilage near their junction	Inf aspect of clavicle in the mid 3rd	Protraction Depression	Branch from brachial plexus (sup trunk)	Thoracoacromial a.
Serratus Anterior	Ext surfaces of ribs 1 to 9	Ant aspect of med border of scapula from sup to inf angle	Protraction Depression ▲ ↻ glen fossa	Long thoracic n.	Lat thoracic a.
Subscapularis	Mid 2/3 subscapular fossa; inf 2/3 groove on axillary	Lesser tubercle of humerus	Med ↻ & / Abd & add	Subscapular n.	Circumflex scapular a.

Muscle	Origin	Insertion	Action	Nerve	Artery
Shoulder/Elbow					
Supraspinatus	Mid 2/3 supraspina-tous fossa	Sub impression of greater tubercle of humerus	Abd Lat ↻ (weak) ↺ (weak)	Suprascapular n.	Suprascapular a.
Infraspinatus	Med 2/3 infraspinatus fossa	Mid impression of greater tubercle of humerus	Lat ↻ Abd & add	Suprascapular n.	Suprascapular a.
Teres Minor	Dorsal surface of axillary border of scapula	Inf impression of greater tubercle of humerus distal to inf impression	Lat ↻ Add	Branch of axillary n.	Post humeral circumflex a.
Teres Major	Oval area on dorsal surface of inf angle of scapula	Crest of lesser tubercle of humerus	Add ↺ / shoulder Med ↻	Lower subscapular n.	Circumflex scapular a.
Deltoideus	Ant border & sup surface of lat 3rd of clavicle; lat margin & sup surface of acromium; inf lip post border scapular spine	Deltoid prominence on mid of lat body of humerus	Abd shoulder ↺ / shoulder ↺ / shoulder Med & lat ↻	Axillary n. from brachial plexus	Post humeral circumflex a.
Shoulder/Elbow					
Triceps Brachii	Long head: infraglenoid tuberosity of scapula;	Post proximal surface of olecranon	↺ / elbow ↺ / shoulder	Branches radial n.	Profunda brachii a.

Muscle	Origin	Insertion	Action	Nerve	Artery
Forearm/Wrist					
Triceps Brachii (*continued*)	Lat head: post surface of humerus; Med head: post surface of humerus distal to radial groove		Add shoulder		Inf ulnar collateral a.
Brachialis	Distal 1/2 of ant-aspect of humerus	Tuberosity of ulna; rough depression on ant surface of coronoid process	✓elbow	Musculocutaneous n. Radial & med n.	Brachial a.
Biceps Brachii	Short head: apex of coracoid process; Long head: supraglenoid tuberosity at sup margin of glenoid	Rough post portion tuberosity of radius	✓ shoulder ✓ elbow Supination	Musculocutaneous n.	Brachial a.
Coracobrachialis	Apex of coracoid process	Impression at med surface & border of humerus	✓ shoulder Add shoulder	Musculocutaneous n.	Brachial a.
Forearm/Wrist Pronator Teres	Humeral head: proximal to med epicondyle of humerus; Ulnar head: med side of coronoid process of ulna	Rough impression at mid of lat surface of radius	Pronation	Median n.	Inf ulnar collateral a.

Muscle	Origin	Insertion	Action	Nerve	Artery
Forearm/Wrist					
Flexor Carpi Radialis	Med epicondyle of humerus	Base of 2nd metacarpal bone	↓ wrist Radial ↓	Median n.	Radial a.
Palmaris Longus	Med epicondyle of humerus	Palmar aponeurosis	↓ wrist	Median n.	Volar interosseous a.
Flexor Carpi Ulnaris	Humeral head: med epicondyle of humerus; Ulnar head: med margin olecranon; proximal 2/3 dorsal border of ulna	Pisiform bone	↓ wrist Add wrist	Ulnar n.	Ulnar a.
Flexor Digitorum Superficialis	Humeral head: med epicondyle of humerus; Ulnar head: med side of coronoid process; Radial head: oblique line of radius	Divides into 4 tendons which are inserted into the sides of the 2nd phalanx	↓ PIPs ↓ MCPs ↓ wrist	Median n.	Ulnar a.
Flexor Digitorum Profundus	Proximal 3/4 of volar & med surfaces of body of ulnar	Bases of last phalanges	↓ DIPs ↓ PIPs ↓ MCPs ↓ wrist	Palmar interosseous n. from median n. Branch of ulnar n.	Ulnar a. Volar interosseous a.
Flexor Pollicis Longus	Grooved volar surface of body of the radius	Base of distal phalanx of the thumb	↓ IP digit I ↓ MCP digit I ↓ & add wrist	Palmar interosseous n. from median n.	Radial a.

Forearm/Wrist

Muscle	Origin	Insertion	Action	Nerve	Artery
Pronator Quadratus	Pronator ridge on distal part of palmar surface of body of ulna; med part of palmar surface of distal 1/4 of ulna	Distal 1/4 of lat border & palmar surface of body of the radius	Pronation	Palmar interosseous n. from median n.	Ulnar & radial a.
Brachioradialis	Proximal 2/3 of lat supracondylar ridge of humerus	Lat side of base of styloid process of radius	✓ elbow	Branch of radial n.	Radial a.
Extensor Carpi Radialis Longus	Distal 1/3 lat supracondylar ridge of humerus	Dorsal surface of base of 2nd metacarpal bone—radial side	/ extension Abd wrist	Radial n.	Radial a.
Extensor Carpi Radialis Brevis	Lat epicondyle of humerus	Dorsal surface of base of 3rd metacarpal bone—radial side	/ wrist Abd wrist	Radial n.	Radial a.
Extensor Carpi Ulnaris	Lat epicondyle of humerus	Prominent tubercle on ulnar side of base of metacarpal V	/ wrist Add wrist	Deep radial n.	Ulnar a.
Extensor Digitorum	Lat epicondyle of humerus	2nd & 3rd phalanges of fingers; dorsal surface of distal phalanx	/ PIPs & DIPs; / MCPs / wrist	Deep radial n.	Ulnar a.
Extensor Digiti Minimi	Common extensor tendon	Expansion of ext digitorum tendon on	/ PIPs, DIPs & MCP digit V	Deep radial n.	Ulnar a.

Hand

Muscle	Origin	Insertion	Action	Nerve	Artery
Anconeus	Separate tendon from dorsal part of lat epicondyle of humerus	Side of olecranon; proximal 1/4 of dorsal surface of body of ulna	/ elbow	Radial n.	Ulnar a.
Abductor Pollicis Longus	Lat part of dorsal surface of body of ulna	Radial side of base of 1st metacarpal bone	Abd IP, MCP of digit I Abd wrist	Deep radial n.	Radial a.
Extensor Pollicis Brevis	Dorsal surface of body of radius distal to that muscle & interosseous membrane	Base of 1st phalanx of thumb	/ IP, MCP of digit I / wrist	Deep radial n.	Radial a.
Extensor Pollicis Longus	Lat part of mid 1/3 of dorsal surface of body of ulna distal to origin of abductor pollicis longus	Base of last phalanx of thumb	/ IP, MCP of digit I / wrist	Deep radial n.	Radial a.
Extensor Indicis	Dorsal surface of body of ulna below origin of extensor pollicis longus	Joins ulnar side of tendon of extensor digitorum	/ & add of IP, MCP digit II	Deep radial n.	Radial a.
Supinator	Lat epicondyle of humerus from ridge of ulna	Lat edge of radial tuberosity & oblique line of radius & med surface of radius posteriorly	Supination	Deep radial n.	Radial a.

Muscle	Origin	Insertion	Action	Nerve	Artery
Hip					
Abductor Pollicis Brevis	Transverse carpal ligament, tuberosity of scaphoid, ridge of trapezium	Radial side of base of 1st phalanx thumb	Abd thumb	Median n.	Radial a.
Opponens Pollicis	Ridge of trapezium	Length of metacarpal bone of thumb on radial side	Abd thumb ✓ thumb Med ⤴	Median n.	Radial a.
Flexor Pollicis Brevis	Distal ridge of trapezium; ulnar side of 1st metacarpal	Radial side of base of proximal phalanx of thumb; ulnar side of base of 1st phalanx	✓ thumb Add thumb	Median & ulnar n.	Radial a.
Adductor Pollicis	Capitale bone, bases of 2nd & 3rd metacarpals	Ulnar side of base of proximal phalanx of thumb	Add thumb	Deep palmar branch of ulnar n.	Ulnar n.
Palmaris Brevis	Tendinous fasciculi from palmar aponeurosis	Skin on ulnar border of palm of hand	Draws skin mid palm	Ulnar n.	Superficial ulnar a.
Abductor Digiti Minimi	Pisiform bone	Ulnar side of base of 1st phalanx of digit V	Abd digit V ✓ proximal phalanx	Ulnar n.	Ulnar a.
Flexor Digiti Minimi Brevis	Convex surface of hamulus of hamate bone	Ulnar side of base of 1st phalanx of digit V	✓ digit V	Ulnar n.	Ulnar a.

Muscle	Origin	Insertion	Action	Nerve	Artery
Hip					
Opponens Digiti Minimi	Convexity of hamulus of hamate bone	Length of metacarpal bone of digit V along ulnar margin	Abd digit V ↙ digit V Med ↗ V	Ulnar n.	Ulnar a.
Lumbricals	Originate from the profundus tendons 1 & 2: radials sides & palmar surfaces of tendons of digits II & III; 3: contiguous sides of mid & ring fingers; 4: contiguous sides of tendons of ring & little finger	Tendinous expansion of extensor digitorum	✓ MCPs / PIPs & DIPs	1 & 2: median n. 3 & 4: ulnar n.	Median a. Ulnar a.
Interosseous Dorsales	2 heads from adjacent sides of metacarpal bone; all from	Bases of 1st phalanx	Abd—midline (digit III)	Deep palmar branch n.	Ulnar a.
Interossei	entire length of metacarpal bones	Side of base of 1st phalanx	Add—midline (digit III) ✓ MCPs / PIPs & DIPs	Deep palmar branch n.	Ulnar a.
Hip					
Psoas Major (Iliopsoas)	Ventral surface of bases and caudal borders of transverse process of	Lesser trochanter of femur	✓ hip ↙ spine in lumbar region	2nd & 3rd lumbar n.	Lumbar branch of iliolumbar a.

Muscle	Origin	Insertion	Action	Nerve	Artery
Hip/Thigh					
Psoas Major (Iliopsoas) *(continued)*	lumbar spine; sides and corresponding intervertebral disks of last thoracic and all lumbar vertebrae				
Psoas Minor (Iliopsoas)	Vertebral margins of T12 & L1, & corresponding disks	Pectineal line; iliopectineal eminence	↘ spine in lumbar region	1st & 2nd lumbar n.	Lumbar branch of iliolumbar a.
Iliacus (Iliopsoas)	Upper 2/3 of iliac fossa; iliac crest	Lesser trochanter of femur	↘ at hip	Femoral n. (muscular branches)	Lumbar branch of iliolumbar a.
Tensor Fasciae Latae (TFL)	Ant part of outer lip of iliac crest; ant border of ilium	Lat part of fascia lata at junction of proximal & mid thirds of thigh (proximal end of iliotibial band)	Tenses TFL ↘ at hip Abd at hip Int ↻ at hip	Sup gluteal n.	Sup gluteal a.
Gluteus Maximus	Post gluteal line; dorsal surface of sacrum & coccyx	Gluteal tuberosity; lat part of TFL at junction of proximal and mid thirds of thigh (proximal end of iliotibial band)	↘ at hip Add at hip Ext ↻ at hip ↘ lower spine	Inf gluteal n.	Inf gluteal a.

Muscle	Origin	Insertion	Action	Nerve	Artery
Leg					
Gluteus Medius	Outer surface of ilium from iliac crest & post gluteal line above to ant gluteal line below	Lat surface of greater trochanter	Abd at hip Int ↻ at hip	Sup gluteal n.	Sup gluteal a.
Piriformis	Pelvic surface of sacrum between ant sacral foramina & margin of greater sciatic foramen	Upper border of greater trochanter of femur	Ext ↻ at hip Abd at hip	1st & 2nd sacral n.	Sup gluteal a.
Obturator Internus	Margins of obturator foramen; pelvic surface of hip bone; post & sup obturator foramen	Med surface of greater trochanter	Ext ↻ at hip Abd at hip	Obturator n. to obturator internus & gemellus sup	Obturator a. Sup gluteal a.
Gemellus Superior	Outer surface of ischial spine	Med surface of greater trochanter	Ext ↻ at hip	Obturator n. to obturator internus & gemellus sup	Obturator a. Sup gluteal a.
Gemellus Inferior	Upper part of ischial tuberosity	Med surface of greater trochanter	Ext ↻ at hip	Obturator n. to quadratus femoris & gemellus inf	Sup gluteal a.
Quadratus Femoris	Lat margin of ischial tuberosity	Quadrate tubercle of femur; linea quadrata	Add at hip Ext ↻ at hip	Obturator n. to quadratus femoris & gemellus inf	Sup gluteal a.
Obturator Externus	Outer margin of obturator foramen	Trochanteric fossa of femur	Add at hip Ext ↻ at hip	Post branch of obturator n.	Obturator a.

Muscle	Origin	Insertion	Action	Nerve	Artery
Leg/Foot					
Sartorius	Ant-sup iliac spine; upper half of iliac notch	Upper part of med surface of tibia	✓ at hip; Ext ↻ at hip; ✓ at knee; Abd hip (weak)	Muscular branches of femoral n.	Femoral a.
Quadriceps Femoris Rectus Femoris	Ant-inf iliac spine	Tibial Tuberosity	/ at knee; ✓ at hip	Muscular branches of femoral n.	Femoral a.
Vastus Lateralis	Lat aspect of the shaft of the femur	Tibial Tuberosity	/ at knee	Muscular branches of femoral n.	Femoral a.
Vastus Medialis	Med aspect of the shaft of the femur	Tibial Tuberosity	/ at knee; draws patella medially	Muscular branches of femoral n.	Femoral a.
Vastus Intermedius	Ant aspect of the shaft of the femur	Tibial Tuberosity	/ at knee	Muscular branches of femoral n.	Femoral a.
Gracilis	Lower 1/2 of pubic symphysis; upper 1/2 of pubic arch	Proximal part of med surface of tibia	✓ at knee; Int ↻ at knee; Add at hip	Ant branch of obturator n.	Med femoral circumflex a. (ascending)
Pectineus	Pubic pectineal line & an area of bone ant to it	Line leading from the lesser trochanter to the linea aspera	Add at hip; ✓ at hip; Int ↻ hip	Muscular branches of femoral & obturator n.	Med femoral circumflex

Muscle	Origin	Insertion	Action	Nerve	Artery
Leg/Foot					
Adductor Longus	Ant portion of pubis in angle between crest & symphysis	Mid part of linea aspera	Add at hip ↗ at hip	Ant branch of obturator n.	Profunda femoris a.
Adductor Brevis	Ext surface of inf ramus of pubis	Proximal part of linea aspera	Add at hip ↗ at hip	Ant branch of obturator n.	Mid femoral circumflex a.
Adductor Magnus	Pubic arch & ischial tuberosity	Oblique line along entire shaft of the femur	Add at hip ↗ hip (upper) ↘ hip (lower)	Post branch of obturator & sciatic n.	Profunda femoris & med femoris circumflex a.
Biceps Femoris	Long head: from ischial tuberosity; Short head: lat lip of linea aspera; lat supra-condylar line of femur	Head of fibula, lat condyle of tibia, deep fascia on lat side of leg	↗ at knee ↘ at hip Ext↻ knee (semiflexed)	Sciatic n. tibial branch to long head; peroneal branch to short head	Profunda femoris a.
Semitendinous	Upper & mid impression of ischial tuberosity (with tendon of the biceps femoris)	Proximal part of ant border & med surface of the tibia	↗ at knee ↘ at hip Int↺ knee (semiflexed)	Sciatic n.	Perforating branch profunda femoris a.
Semimembranous	Proximal & lat facet of ischial tuberosity	Med-post surface of med condyle of tibia	↗ at knee ↘ at hip Int↺ knee (semiflexed)	Sciatic n.	Perforating branch profunda femoris a.

Muscle	Origin	Insertion	Action	Nerve	Artery
Foot					
Tibialis Anterior	Lat surface of shaft of tibia; med aspect of fibula; ant interosseus membrane	Med & plantar surface of med cuniform bone; base of 1st metatarsal bone	Dorsiflexion inversion	Deep peroneal n.	Ant tibial a.
Popliteus	Lat condyle of femur	Triangular area on post surface of tibia above sdeal line	✓ at knee Int ↻ at knee	Tibial n. (med & int popliteal)	Post tibial a.
Leg/Foot					
Extensor Hallucis Longus	Lat surface of shaft of tibia; med aspect of fibula; ant interosseous membrane	Base of distal phalanx of great toe	/ MTP & IP Dorsiflexion	Deep peroneal n. (ant tibial)	Ant tibial a.
Extensor Digitorum Longus (EDL)	Lat surface of shaft of tibia; med aspect of fibula; ant - interosseous membrane	Dorsal surface of mid & distal phalanges of lat 4 digits	/ IPs digits II to V Dorsiflexion	Deep peroneal n. (ant tibial)	Ant tibial a.
Extensor Digitorum Brevis (EDB)	Proximal & lat surface of calcaneus; lat talo-calcaneal ligament	1st tendon dorsal surface of base of proximal phalanx of hallux; other 3 tendons lat sides of tendons of EDL	/ IPs	Deep peroneal n.	Ant tibial a.

Foot

Muscle	Origin	Insertion	Action	Nerve	Artery
Flexor Digitorum Longus	Post surface of shaft of tibia; post aspect of fibula; post interosseous membrane	Plantar surface of base of distal phalanx of lat 4 digits	✓ digits II to V Plantar-flexion	Tibial n. (med & int popliteal)	Post tibial a.
Flexor Hallucis Longus	Post surface of shaft of tibia; post aspect of fibula; post interosseous membrane	Base of distal phalanx of hallux	✓ digit I Plantarflexion	Tibial n. (med & int popliteal)	Post tibial a.
Tibialis Posterior	Post surface of shaft of tibia; post aspect of fibula; post interosseous membrane	Tuberosity of navicular; plantar surface of cuniform bones; plantar surface of base of 2nd, 3rd & 4th metatarsals, cuboid, sustentaculum tali	Plantarflexion Inversion	Tibial n. (med & int popliteal)	Post tibial a.
Peroneus Tertius	Lat surface of shaft of tibia; med aspect of fibula; ant interosseous membrane	Dorsal surface of base of 5th metatarsal bone	Dorsiflexion Eversion	Deep peroneal n. (ant tibial)	Ant tibial a.
Peroneus Longus	Lat condyle of tibia; head & upper 2/3 of lat surface of fibula	Lat side of med cuniform bone, base of 1st metatarsal bone	Plantarflexion Eversion	Superficial peroneal n. (musculocutaneous)	Peroneal a.

Muscle	Origin	Insertion	Action	Nerve	Artery
Foot					
Peroneus Brevis	Lower 2/3 of lat surface of fibula	Lat side of base of 5th metatarsal bone	Plantarflexion Eversion	Superficial peroneal n. (musculocutaneous)	Peroneal a.
Gastrocnemius	Med head: med condyle & adjacent part of femur; capsule of knee; Long head: lat condyle & adjacent part of femur; capsule of knee	Calcaneus by the calcaneal tendon	Plantarflexion ✓ at knee	Tibial n. (med popliteal)	Popliteal a.
Soleus	Post surface of head & proximal 1/3 of shaft of fibula; mid 1/3 of med border of tibia	Calcaneus by the calcaneal tendon	Plantarflexion	Tibial n. (med popliteal)	Post tibial a.
Plantaris	Lat supracondylar line of femur	Med side of post part of calcaneus	Plantarflexion	Tibial n. (med popliteal)	Post tibial a.
Quadratus Plantae	Med head: med surface of calcaneus & med border of long plantar ligament; Lat head: lat border of plantar surface of calcaneus & lat border of long plantar ligament	Attached to tendons of flexor digitorum longus	✓ last IP digits II to V	Lat plantar n.	Lat plantar a.

Muscle	Origin	Insertion	Action	Nerve	Artery
Foot					
Lumbricals (4)	Tendons of flexor digitorum longus	Tendons of EDL & interossei into bases of last phalanges of digits II-V	✓ MP joints / IP joints	Med plantar n. Deep lat plantar n.	Med plantar a.

Key:
✓ flexion
/ extension
↻ rotation
▼ depression, downward, caudal
▲ elevation, upward, cephalic
◆▶ outward, expand
n. = nerve
a. = artery
Lat = lateral
Med = medial
Ext = external
Int = internal
Sup = superior
Inf = inferior

Ant = anterior
Post = posterior
Min = minimal
MTP = metatarsophalangeal
MCP = metacarpophalangeal
IP = interphalangeal
PIP = proximal interphalangeal
DIP = distal interphalangeal
Opp = opposite
Abd = abduction
Add = adduction
Mid = middle

Reprinted with permission from Bottomley J. *Quick Reference Dictionary for Physical Therapy*. Thorofare, NJ: SLACK Incorporated; 2000.

Anatomy—Bones

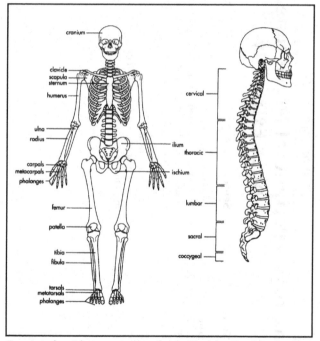

cranium

clavicle
scapula
sternum
humerus

ulna
radius

carpals
metacarpals
phalanges

femur

patella

tibia
fibula

tarsals
metatarsals
phalanges

cervical

ilium
thoracic

ischium

lumbar

sacral

coccygeal

Reprinted with permission from Sladyk K. *OT Student Primer: A Guide to College Success.* Thorofare, NJ: SLACK Incorporated; 1997.

Anatomy—Peripheral Nerve Innervations— Upper Extremity

Peripheral Nerve	Sensory Area	Manual Muscle Test
Axillary (C5 to 6)	Upper deltoid area	Deltoid, teres minor
Musculocutaneous (C5 to 7)	Anterior and lateral upper arm	Biceps brachii
Radial (C5 to T1)	Posterior arm, dorsum of hand	Triceps, wrist extensors
Ulnar (C7 to T1)	Anterior/medial forearm, fourth and fifth fingers	Ulnar flexion, flexor digitorum profundus for last 2 digits
Median (C6 to T1)	Anterior/lateral forearm, palmar thumb, first, second finger, half of third finger	Thenar eminence, pronators

Chen AF, ed.
Quick Reference Dictionary for Orthopedics (pp 268-270).
© 2012 Taylor & Francis Group

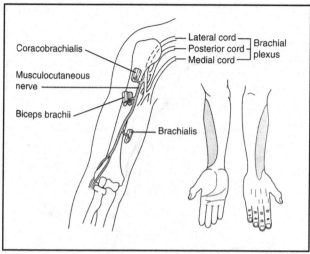

Figure 6-1. Motor and sensory distribution of musculocutaneous nerves. (Reprinted with permission from Magee D. *Orthopedic Physical Assessment.* 3rd ed. Philadelphia, PA: WB Saunders; 1997.)

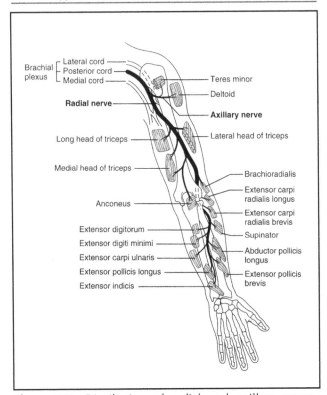

Figure 6-2. Distribution of radial and axillary nerves. (Reprinted with permission from Magee D. *Orthopedic Physical Assessment.* 3rd ed. Philadelphia, PA: WB Saunders; 1997.)

Anatomy—Peripheral Nerve Innervations— Lower Extremity

Peripheral Nerve	Sensory Area	Manual Muscle Test
Femoral	Medial thigh and leg	Quadriceps
Sciatic (common peroneal and tibial)	Posterior thigh and leg	Hamstrings (tibial)
Obturator	Mid anterior thigh	Adductors
Common peroneal	See deep and superficial peroneal	See deep and superficial peroneal
Deep peroneal	Web space between 1st and 2nd toes	Dorsiflexors
Superficial peroneal	Medial dorsal surface of foot	Evertors
Tibial	Posterior leg	Hamstrings and plantar flexors

Chen AF, ed.
Quick Reference Dictionary
for Orthopedics (pp 271-276).

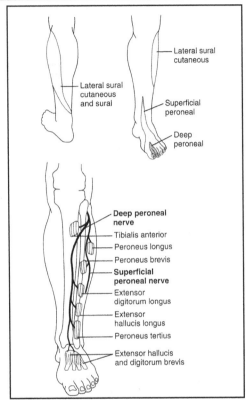

Figure 7-1. Common peroneal nerve. (Reprinted with permission from Magee D. *Orthopedic Physical Assessment.* 3rd ed. Philadelphia, PA: WB Saunders; 1997.)

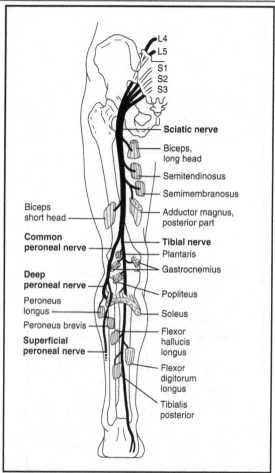

Figure 7-2. Sciatic nerve and its branches. (Reprinted with permission from Magee D. *Orthopedic Physical Assessment*. 3rd ed. Philadelphia, PA: WB Saunders; 1997.)

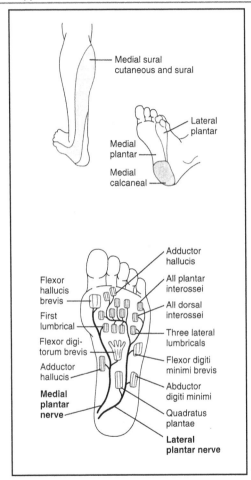

Figure 7-3. Medial and lateral plantar nerves. (Reprinted with permission from Magee D. *Ortho-pedic Physical Assessment.* 3rd ed. Philadelphia, PA: WB Saunders; 1997.)

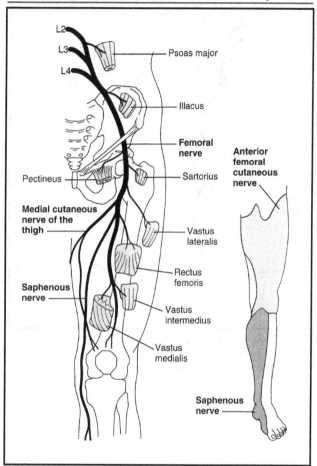

Figure 7-4. Femoral nerve. (Reprinted with permission from Magee D. *Orthopedic Physical Assessment.* 3rd ed. Philadelphia, PA: WB Saunders; 1997.)

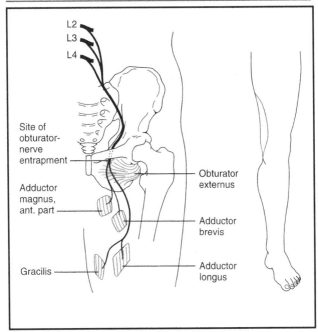

Figure 7-5. Obturator nerve. (Reprinted with permission from Magee D. *Orthopedic Physical Assessment.* 3rd ed. Philadelphia, PA: WB Saunders; 1997.)

Nerve Root Assessment—Upper Extremity

Nerve Root	Dermatome	Myotome	Reflex
C4	Top shoulder and neck	Elevate shoulders	—
C5	Lateral upper arm, shoulder	Shoulder abduction	Biceps
C6	Lateral arm, thumb	Elbow flexion/wrist extension	Brachioradialis
C7	Middle finger, posterior middle arm	Elbow extension/wrist flexion	Triceps
C8	Medial hand	Finger flexion	—
T1	Medial elbow	Finger abduction/adduction	—

APPENDIX 9

Nerve Root Assessment—Lower Extremity

Nerve Root	Dermatome	Myotome	Reflex
L1	Anterior upper thigh, lateral hip	Hip flexion	—
L2	Anterior mid-thigh	Hip flexion, knee extension	Patella
L3	Lower anterior medial thigh (area of vastus medialis oblique [vmol])	Knee extension	Patella
L4	Anterior/medial leg	Dorsiflexion (heel walking)	Patella
L5	Anterior/lateral leg	Knee flexion, great toe extension	Tibialis posterior
S1	Lateral ankle	Knee flexion, plantarflexion (toe walking)	Achilles
S2	Posterior superior lower leg	—	—

Chen AF, ed.
Quick Reference Dictionary for Orthopedics (p 278).
© 2012 Taylor & Francis Group

Dermatomes

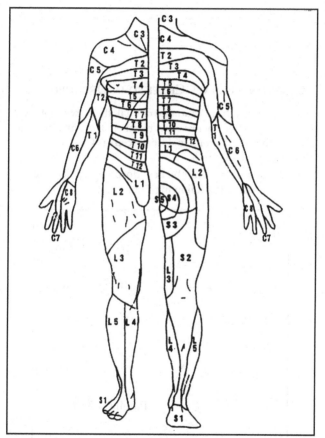

Reflexes

COMMON REFLEXES CHECKED IN ORTHOPEDICS

- As you go from caudal to cranial, the nerve root level being tested increases in number. The ankle is S1 to 2, the patella is L3 to 4, the biceps is C5 to 6, and the triceps are C7 to 8.
- These numbers can be best documented and memorized using the following figure:

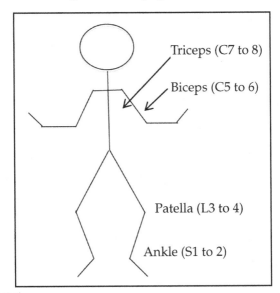

Triceps (C7 to 8)

Biceps (C5 to 6)

Patella (L3 to 4)

Ankle (S1 to 2)

Chen AF, ed.
Quick Reference Dictionary for Orthopedics (pp 280-286).
© 2012 Taylor & Francis Group.

GRADING SCALE

0 = no response; always abnormal
1+ = a slight but definitely present response; may or may not be normal
2+ = a brisk response; normal
3+ = a very brisk response; may or may not be normal
4+ = a tap elicits a repeating reflex (clonus); always abnormal

Deep Tendon Reflexes	Test	Response
Brachioradialis (C5 to 6)	Subject sits with elbow flexed and forearm comfortably resting on surface. Thumb is placed proximally from the radial styloid (on the brachioradialis insertion) and is tapped with a reflex hammer.	Slight wrist extension, radial deviation, supination, and elbow flexion
Biceps (C5 to 6)	Subject sits with elbow flexed and forearm supported. The thumb is placed over the biceps tendon in the antecubital fossa and the thumb is tapped.	Slight elbow flexion
Triceps (C7 to 8)	Subject sits with shoulder abducted and internally rotated, with elbow flexed and supported. The triceps tendon can be palpated proximal to the olecranon and the tendon can be tapped.	Slight elbow extension
Hamstring (L2 to 4)	Subject is placed prone with knee slightly flexed and foot supported. The tendon is palpated posterior to the knee and the tendon is tapped.	Slight knee flexion
Patellar (L2 to 4)	Subject sits with knees flexed and feet unsupported. The patella tendon is palpated inferior to the patella and is tapped.	Knee extension

Deep Tendon Reflexes	Test	Response
Ankle (S1 to 2)	Subject sits with knees flexed and feet unsupported. A hand is placed on the forefoot to hold the foot in neutral. The Achilles tendon is palpated superior to the calcaneus and the tendon is tapped.	Slight plantarflexion
Upper Motor Neuron Reflexes	**Test**	**Response**
Hoffman	Subject's hand is gently flexed at the metacarpo-phalangeal joint. The terminal phalanx or nail of the long finger is tapped or flicked.	Flexion of the terminal phalanx of the thumb is an abnormal response. The response may be normal in young, healthy women who are hyperreflexive.
Abdominal (T7 to 12)	Subject placed supine on examining table. A finger is used to make quick and light strokes across the abdomen from the periphery to the umbilicus. The reflex is tested in all 4 quadrants of the abdomen	Localized contraction of the umbilicus toward the quadrant stimulated is normal

Upper Motor Neuron Reflexes	Test	Response
Babinski (plantar reflex)	Subject sits with feet unsupported and the sole of the foot is stroked with a finger or the bottom of a reflex hammer from the heel to the base of the great toe.	The great toe is extended and the toes fan outwards. This reflex is normal in newborns and is abnormal in individuals greater than 1 year old

Primitive Reflexes	Test	Response
Crossed extension	Subject is supine. Noxious stimulus applied to ball of foot of extremity in extension.	The contralateral lower extremity flexes, adducts, and extends Onset: 28 weeks' gestation Integrated: 1 to 2 months of age
Flexor withdrawal	Subject is supine or sitting. Noxious stimulus (pinprick) applied to sole of foot.	The toes extend, foot dorsiflexes, and the entire leg flexes Onset: 28 weeks' gestation Integrated: 1 to 2 months of age

Primitive Reflexes

Primitive Reflexes	Test	Response
Moro/startle	Subject is supine. A sudden or loud noise is made or the head suddenly shifts position.	The legs and head extend and the arms suddenly extend and abduct with palms up and thumbs flexed. The arms adduct and the hands clench into fists. The subject often cries. Onset: birth Integrated: 5 to 6 months of age
Palmar grasp	Subject is supine or sitting and pressure is placed on the palms.	The fingers flex Onset: birth Integrated: 4 to 6 months of age
Plantar grasp	Subject is supine and pressure is placed on the metatarsal heads.	The toes flex Onset: 28 weeks' gestation Integrated: 9 months of age
Rooting	The cheek of a subject is stroked.	The head will turn toward the direction of the stroke Onset: birth Integrated: 4 months of age

Primitive Reflexes	Test	Response
Sucking	Item is placed within the subject's mouth.	The subject starts to suck when an object touches the roof of his or her mouth Onset: birth Integrated: 4 months of age
Tonic neck	Subject is supine. The head is turned to one side.	The ipsilateral arm will straighten and the contralateral arm will flex Onset: 1 month of age Integrated: 4 to 5 months of age
Traction	Subject is supine. Grasp forearm and pull from supine into sitting position.	With grasping, the upper extremity flexes Onset: 28 weeks' gestation Integrated: 2 to 5 months of age
Walking/stepping	Subject is held in the air and the feet are brought the close to a flat surface.	The plantar surface of feet will touch the flat surface, which appears as walking Onset: birth Integrated: 6 weeks of age

Muscle Strength Scale
(0 to 5 Scale)

Muscle strength is graded by the Medical Research Council (MRC) Scale, where 0 is the lowest and 5 is the highest. This strength scale can be used to rate each muscle or a group of muscles. It is most useful as a comparative number, as opposed to an absolute number, because one person's grading may differ from another person's. This scale is effective for assessing whether a patient's muscle strength is improving by comparing strength at different time points. The scale is as follows:

0 = No contraction
1 = Trace contraction (fasciculation, no movement of the joint)
2 = Active movement with gravity eliminated
3 = Active movement against gravity
4 = Active movement against resistance
5 = Normal strength, able to overcome full resistance

Normal Joint Ranges of Motion

SPINE RANGE OF MOTION

	Cervical	*Lumbar*
Forward flexion	0 to 45 degrees	0 to 95 degrees
Extension	0 to 50 degrees	0 to 35 degrees
Lateral flexion	0 to 45 degrees	0 to 40 degrees
Rotation	0 to 60 degrees	0 to 35 degrees

UPPER EXTREMITY RANGE OF MOTION

Shoulder

Flexion	0 to 180 degrees
Extension	0 to 60 degrees
Abduction	0 to 180 degrees
Adduction	0 to 75 degrees
Horizontal abduction	0 to 90 degrees
Horizontal adduction	0 to 45 degrees
Internal rotation	0 to 70 to 90 degrees
External rotation	0 to 90 degrees

Elbow and Forearm

Extension to flexion	0 to 150 degrees
Supination	0 to 80 to 90 degrees
Pronation	0 to 80 to 90 degrees

Chen AF, ed.
*Quick Reference Dictionary
for Orthopedics (pp 288-290).*
© 2012 Taylor & Francis Group.

Wrist

Flexion	0 to 80 to 90 degrees
Extension	0 to 70 degrees
Ulnar deviation	0 to 30 to 35 degrees
Radial deviation	0 to 20 degrees

Thumb (first digit)

CM flexion	0 to 15 degrees
CM extension	0 to 20 degrees
MCP flexion	0 to 50 to 90 degrees
MCP extension	0 to 10 degrees
IP flexion	0 to 80 to 110 degrees
IP extension	0 to 10 degrees
Abduction	0 to 70 degrees
Opposition	0 (cm)

Fingers (second through fifth digits)

MCP flexion	0 to 90 degrees
PIP flexion	0 to 100 to 110 degrees
PIP extension	0 to 10 degrees
DIP flexion	0 to 90 to 110 degrees
DIP extension	0 to 10 degrees
Abduction	No norm
Adduction	No norm

LOWER EXTREMITY RANGE OF MOTION

Hip

Flexion	0 to 120 degrees
Extension	0 to 10 degrees
Abduction	0 to 45 degrees
Adduction	0 to 30 degrees
Medial rotation	0 to 45 degrees
Lateral rotation	0 to 45 degrees

Knee

Extension to flexion	0 to 135 to 145 degrees

Ankle to Foot

Dorsiflexion	0 to 20 degrees
Plantarflexion	0 to 45 degrees
Inversion	0 to 30 degrees
Eversion	0 to 20 degrees

Great Toe (first digit)

MTP flexion	0 to 45 degrees
MTP extension	0 to 90 degrees
IP flexion	0 to 90 degrees
IP extension	0 to 70 degrees

Lesser Toes (second through fifth digit)

MTP flexion	0 to 40 degrees
MTP extension	0 to 45 degrees
PIP flexion	0 to 45 degrees
DIP flexion	0 to 70 degrees

MTP = metatarsalphalangeal
DIP = distal interphalangeal
IP = interphalangeal
CM = carpometacarpal
MCP = metacarpophalangeal
PIP = proximal interphalangeal

Aspiration and Injection of and Around Joints

Aspirating and injecting joints are a vital part of orthopedics to deliver intra-articular medication, aspirate fluid, and determine the presence of an open joint injury. For every injection, be sure to maintain sterile technique and use an appropriate needle. A spinal needle may be necessary for deeper joints (hips and shoulders), and the needle should not be smaller than a 21-gauge needle. Joint aspirations should be performed with an 18-gauge needle. When aspirating or injecting a joint, never perform these procedures over erythematous skin.

1. Shoulder (glenohumeral joint, subacromial space, and acromioclavicular joint)

   a. Positioning: The patient should be sitting up with the arm comfortably at the patient's side, allowing the humerus to fall away from the glenoid.

   b. Anterior (Figure 14-1)

      i. The humeral head is palpated and the needle is placed immediately medial to the humeral head to reach the glenohumeral joint.

      ii. To reach the acromioclavicular joint, the clavicle is palpated laterally until there is a slight depression at the junction between the clavicle and the acromion. A needle may be placed on the end of the acromion or the clavicle and "walked" toward the joint until the needle "falls" into the joint.

Chen AF, ed.
*Quick Reference Dictionary
for Orthopedics (pp 291-300).*

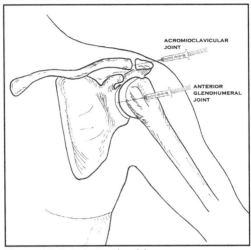

Figure 14-1. Anterior shoulder.

c. Posterior: More common approach (Figure 14-2)

   i. The posterolateral corner of the acromion should be palpated and the "soft spot" 2 cm inferior and 1 cm medial should be palpated (1 finger breadth is approximately 1 cm). The needle should be directed toward the coracoid process, which can be palpated on the anterior aspect of the shoulder. When the capsule of the glenohumeral joint is entered, there will be a "popping" sensation.

   ii. To reach the subacromial space, the needle starts in the same location but is directed approximately 30 degrees cephalad. The needle can be directed superiorly to hit the acromion and then placed immediately below the acromion to enter the subacromial space.

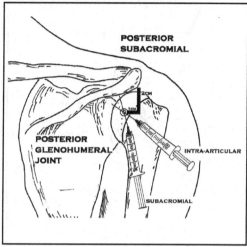

Figure 14-2. Posterior shoulder.

2. Elbow (Figure 14-3)

   a. Positioning: The patient should be seated with the elbow flexed and forearm supported. For medial epicondylitis, the arm should be abducted and the forearm supinated. For lateral epicondylitis, the arm should be adducted and the forearm pronated.

   b. Olecranon fossa: The anatomic landmarks for elbow arthrocentesis are the lateral epicondyle of the humerus, the radial head, and the lateral olecranon. These structures form a triangle, and in the middle of this triangle there should be a "soft spot" where the needle should be placed. The needle should enter the joint easily; if not, the needle may need to be redirected.

   c. Lateral epicondyle

      i. This injection is used to treat lateral epicondylitis (ie, tennis elbow).

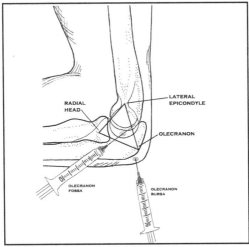

Figure 14-3. Elbow

    ii. The tender spot can be palpated and is often proximal to the lateral epicondyle. Once identified, the needle should be inserted in this area through the extensor carpi radialis brevis (ECRB) onto bone and then withdrawn 1 to 2 mm to permit injection.

d. Medial epicondyle

    i. This injection is used to treat medial epicondylitis (ie, golfer's elbow).

    ii. The tender spot can be palpated medially, and the needle should be inserted in this area onto bone. The needle should be withdrawn 1 to 2 mm to permit injection.

e. Olecranon

    i. This injection is used to treat olecranon bursitis.

    ii. Olecranon bursas should be palpable and can be found directly over the proximal ulna. The needle should be introduced directly into the bursa to aspirate fluid and inject corticosteroids as needed.

3. Wrist (Figure 14-4)

   a. Positioning: The patient's hand should be placed prone on a flat surface so that the dorsal surface is easily accessible.

   b. Radiocarpal joint

      i. Radial: The radiocarpal joint can be accessed between the third and fourth extensor tendon compartments, approximately 1 cm distal to the Lister tubercle. The thumb can be abducted to allow easier access to the radiocarpal joint.

      ii. Ulna: The distal ulna can be palpated and the needle can be directed volarly and radially.

   c. Intercarpal joint: The intercarpal joint is difficult to access. The needle may be inserted approximately 2 cm distal from the Lister tubercle to enter this joint.

   d. Distal radioulnar joint: The area between the fourth and fifth extensor tendon compartment can be palpated, which is immediately radial from the ulna. A needle can be inserted within this compartment.

4. Hip (Figure 14-5)

   a. Positioning: The patient should be placed supine on an examination table. This injection is often performed under fluoroscopic guidance.

   b. Anterolateral: The landmarks are the femoral artery and the greater trochanter. The femoral artery should be palpated and marked, as well as the tip of the greater trochanter. For this approach, a line is drawn from the intersection of the femoral vessels and the inguinal ligament to the greater trochanter, and the needle is inserted at the halfway point. The needle is directed 45 degrees cranial and abducted to follow the femoral neck. The needle is advanced past the femoral neck and into the capsule. A "pop" should be felt. Fluoroscopy is used

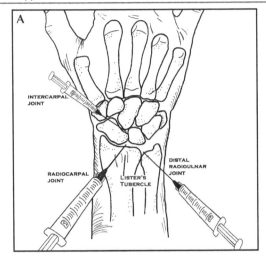

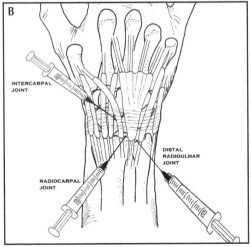

Figure 14-4. (A) Wrist showing bones. (B) Wrist showing tendons.

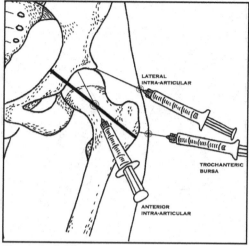

Figure 14-5. Hip.

to confirm needle placement with an air or contrast arthrogram.

c. Lateral: The landmarks are the same for this approach, but the needle is placed proximal to the tip of the greater trochanter and directed at the femoral head and neck junction. The needle is angled approximately 20 degrees cephalad to follow the anteversion of the femoral neck. Once a "pop" is felt when the capsule is entered, fluoroscopy is used to confirm placement.

d. Greater trochanter: This approach is used to treat greater trochanteric bursitis and fluoroscopy is not necessary. The patient is placed in a lateral position and the greater trochanter is palpated. The most tender location is found and the needle is directed toward the greater trochanter directly to bone. The needle should be pulled back 1 to 2 mm where the injection should be given.

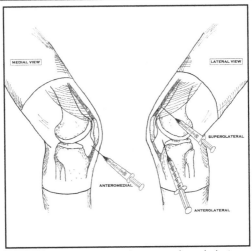

Figure 14-6. Knee, lateral view and medial view.

5. Knee (Figure 14-6)

   a. Positioning: The patient may be placed supine for the superolateral approach. For the anteromedial and anterolateral approach, the patient should be sitting upright with the knees flexed.

   b. Superolateral: Most common approach: The patient's patella is palpated and tilted medially. The needle enters the joint in the suprapatellar pouch, posterior to the proximal pole of the patella and perpendicular to the femur. If the needle is within the joint, there should be minimal resistance. This approach is beneficial for effusions.

   c. Anteromedial: With the knee flexed, the anteromedial location can be palpated immediately medial to the patella tendon at the inferior pole of the patella. The needle should enter the joint with ease and should be directed approximately 30 degrees caudal and 30 degrees laterally toward the trochanteric notch. This approach is beneficial for injections.

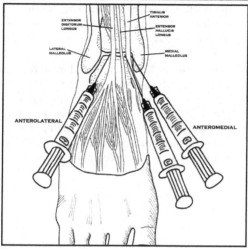

Figure 14-7. Ankle.

    d. Anterolateral: With the knee flexed, the anterolateral location can be palpated immediately lateral to the patella tendon at the inferior pole of the patella. The needle should enter the joint with ease and should be directed approximately 30 degrees caudal and 30 degrees medially toward the trochanteric notch.

6. Ankle (Figure 14-7)

    a. Positioning: The patient should be placed supine on an examination table or with the knee flexed and the foot plantarflexed against a flat surface at approximately 45 degrees.

    b. Anteromedial: The tibialis anterior (TA) and extensor hallucis longus (EHL) tendons are identified. The needle can be inserted between the medial border of the EHL and the lateral border of the TA. The needle can also be inserted medial to the TA, between the TA and the medial malleolus. In both approaches, the needle should be directed laterally and inserted approximately 45 to 60 degrees in an oblique manner to avoid damaging the cartilage surface.

c. Anterolateral: The lateral border of the extensor digitorum longus and the lateral malleolus are identified. The needle is inserted within this space, approx-imately 45 to 60 degrees in an oblique manner medially to avoid damaging the cartilage surface. This approach avoids injury to the dorsalis pedis vessels and the deep peroneal nerve.

Common Fracture Classifications

There are multiple ways used to classify fractures. Some classification schemes are based on fracture pattern and others are based on fracture location. This appendix contains common fracture classifications used in orthopedics.

ARBEITSGEMEINSCHAFT FÜR OSTEOSYNTHESEFRAGEN FRACTURE CLASSIFICATION

The Arbeitsgemeinschaft für Osteosynthesefragen (AO) fracture classification is an alphanumeric classification scheme based on the location and the severity of a fracture. The first number describes the bone where the fracture is located.

1. Humerus
2. Radius/ulna
3. Femur/patella
4. Tibia/fibula
5. Spine
6. Pelvis/acetabulum
7. Hand
8. Foot
9. Craniomaxillofacial

The second number specifies the location of the fracture by dividing long bones into segments.

Chen AF, ed.
*Quick Reference Dictionary
for Orthopedics (pp 301-315).*

1. Proximal
2. Diaphyseal
3. Distal
4. Malleolar

The next part of the classification is a letter that is used to describe the morphology of the fracture. For diaphyseal fractures, the classification is as follows:

A. Simple fracture with a single fragment
B. Multiple fragments that can be reduced
C. Comminuted fracture with multiple fragments that may be impossible to reconstruct

For distal or proximal fractures with intra-articular injury, the classification is as follows:

A. Extra-articular
B. Partial articular
C. Complete articular

The last number ranges from 1 to 3 and describes fracture patterns (eg, spiral, oblique, transverse, wedge, depression, split depression) depending on the location of the fracture, and it describes concomitant injuries (if a single or both bones are fractured or if the joint is dislocated).

Examples:
- Simple spiral diaphyseal humerus fracture: 12-A1
- Simple lateral and medial malleolar fractures: 44-A2

UPPER EXTREMITIES

Clavicle Fractures

- Classification: Allman
- Groups: 3
  o Group I: Middle one-third fracture (most common)
  o Group II: Distal one-third fracture
  o Group III: Proximal one-third fracture

Glenoid Fractures

- Classification: Ideberg and Goss
- Types: 6
  - Type I: Anterior glenoid avulsion fracture
  - Type II: Inferior glenoid fracture
    * Type IIA: Transverse inferior glenoid fracture
    * Type IIB: Oblique inferior glenoid fracture
  - Type III: Superior glenoid fracture
  - Type IV: Transverse glenoid fracture through scapular body
  - Type V: Inferior glenoid and scapular body fracture
  - Type VI: Comminuted glenoid fracture

Proximal Humerus Fractures

- Classification: Neer
  - Fracture classification defined as 45-degree angulation and 1-cm displacement
- Parts: 4
  - Part 1: Greater tuberosity
  - Part 2: Lesser tuberosity
  - Part 3: Shaft (anatomic neck versus surgical neck)
  - Part 4: Head

Distal Humerus/Intercondylar Humerus Fractures (T-type)

- Classification: Riseborough and Radin
- Types: 4
  - Type I: Nondisplaced
  - Type II: Slight displacement of condyles with no rotation
  - Type III: Displacement of condyles with rotation
  - Type IV: Severe comminution of the articular surfaces

Coronoid Process Fracture

- Classification: Regan and Morrey
- Types: 3
  - Type I: Avulsion of the tip of the coronoid process
  - Type II: Fracture of the coronoid process involving less than 50%
  - Type III: Fracture of the coronoid process involving greater than 50%

Olecranon Fracture

- Classification: Mayo
- Types: 3
  - Type I: Nondisplaced or minimally displaced olecranon fracture
    * Type IA: No comminution
    * Type IB: Comminution
  - Type II: Displacement of the proximal fragment with no elbow instability
    * Type IIA: No comminution
    * Type IIB: Comminution
  - Type III: Olecranon fracture with displacement and elbow instability

Radial Head Fractures

- Classification: Mason
- Types: 4
  - Type I: Nondisplaced fracture
  - Type II: Fracture involving a portion of the head (depression, angulation, or impaction)
  - Type III: Comminuted fracture involving the entire head
  - Type IV: Comminuted fracture involving the entire head with elbow dislocation

Monteggia Fracture

- Classification: Bado
- Types: 4
  - Type I: Extension: Anterior dislocation of the radial head; ulnar shaft fracture at any level with anterior angulation
  - Type II: Flexion: Posterior/posterolateral dislocation of the radial head; ulnar shaft fracture with posterior angulation
  - Type III: Lateral: Lateral/anterolateral dislocation of the radial head; ulnar metaphysis fracture
  - Type IV: Combination: Radial shaft fracture (proximal one-third) with anterior dislocation of the radial head; ulnar shaft fracture at the same level with anterior angulation

Distal Radius Fractures (Eponyms)

- Colles fracture: Distal radius fracture with dorsal displacement, apex volar, radial shift, and shortening
- Smith fracture: Distal radius fracture with volar displacement and apex dorsal
- Barton fracture: Distal radius fracture of the dorsal or volar lip of the radius
- Radial styloid fracture: An avulsion fracture of the radial styloid (also known as a chauffeur fracture)
- Malone fracture:
  - Parts: 5
    * Dorsal lunate fossa
    * Central lunate fossa
    * Volar lunate fossa
    * Radial styloid
    * Radial shaft

Scaphoid Fractures

- Classification: Anatomic

- Types: 3
  - Type A: Distal pole fracture
    * Type A1: Extra-articular fracture of the distal pole
    * Type A2: Intra-articular fracture of the distal pole
  - Type B: Middle third (waist) fracture
  - Type C: Proximal pole fracture

LOWER EXTREMITIES

Pelvis Fractures

- Classification: Young and Burgess
- Types: 4
  - Lateral compression (LC): Transverse fractures of pubic rami
    * LC I: Sacral compression with rami fracture
    * LC II: Iliac wing (crescent) and rami fracture with posterior sacroiliac (SI) ligament disruption
    * LC III: LC I or II fracture with contralateral anteroposterior compression (APC) III fracture (also known as windswept pelvis)
  - APC: Longitudinal rami fractures and symphyseal diastasis
    * APC I: Less than 2.5-cm pubic diastasis fracture
    * APC II: Greater than 2.5-cm pubic diastasis fracture and widened SI joint. Disruption of anterior SI, sacrospinous and sacrotuberous ligaments, intact posterior SI ligament
    * APC III: Complete pubic symphysis and SI joint disruption (unstable)
  - Vertical shear (VS): Vertical displacement due to anterior and posterior pelvis injury (unstable)
  - Combined mechanism (CM): Most often a combination of LC and VS

Acetabular Fractures

- Classification: Judet-Letournel (commonly known as Letournel)

- Elementary fractures: 5
  - Posterior wall
  - Posterior column
  - Anterior wall
  - Anterior column
  - Transverse
- Associated fractures: 5
  - T-shaped
  - Posterior column and posterior wall
  - Transverse and posterior wall
  - Anterior column/posterior hemitransverse
  - Both columns

Hip Dislocations

- Classification: Thompson and Epstein classification (posterior)
- Types: 5
  - Type I: Simple dislocation
  - Type II: Dislocation with large posterior wall fracture fragment
  - Type III: Dislocation with comminuted posterior wall fracture fragments
  - Type IV: Dislocation with acetabular floor fracture
  - Type V: Dislocation with femoral head fracture
- Classification: Epstein classification (anterior)
- Types: 2
  - Type I: Superior dislocation
    * Type IA: No additional fractures
    * Type IB: Concomitant femoral head fracture
    * Type IC: Concomitant acetabular fracture
  - Type II: Inferior dislocation
    * Type IIA: No additional fractures
    * Type IIB: Concomitant femoral head fracture
    * Type IIC: Concomitant acetabular fracture

Femoral Head Fractures

- Classification: Pipkin
- Types: 4
  - Type I: Hip dislocation with femoral head fracture inferior to the fovea

- Type II: Hip dislocation with femoral head fracture superior to the fovea
- Type III: Type I or II injury with concomitant femoral neck fracture
- Type IV: Type I or II injury with concomitant acetabular rim fracture

Femoral Neck Fractures

- Classification: Anatomic
- Types: 3
  - Subcapital: Immediately inferior to the femoral head
  - Transcervical: In the mid-portion of the femoral neck
  - Basicervical: At the base of the femoral neck
- Classification: Garden
- Types: 4
  - Type I: Valgus impacted
  - Type II: Complete fracture without displacement
  - Type III: Complete fracture with partial displacement (the trabecular pattern of bone does not line up with the acetabulum)
  - Type IV: Complete fracture with complete displacement (the trabecular pattern of bone is parallel with the acetabulum)
- Classification: Pauwel (based on the angle of the fracture from the horizontal plane)
- Types: 3
  - Type I < 30 degrees
  - Type II < 50 degrees
  - Type III < 70 degrees

Subtrochanteric Femur Fractures

- Classification: Fielding (based on the fracture line with reference to the lesser trochanter)
- Types: 3
  - Type I: At the level of the lesser trochanter
  - Type II: Less than 2.5 cm below the level of the lesser trochanter

  ○ Type III: 2.5 to 5 cm below the level of the lesser trochanter

Periprosthetic Femur Fracture

- Classification: Vancouver
- Types: 3
  ○ Type A: Trochanteric fracture
  ○ Type B: Around the stem
    * Type B1: Stable prosthesis
    * Type B2: Unstable prosthesis, good bone
    * Type B3: Unstable prosthesis, poor bone
  ○ Type C: Distal to the stem

Femoral Shaft Fractures

- Classification: Winquist and Hansen
- Types: 4
  ○ Type I: Minimal or no comminution
  ○ Type II: Cortices of both fragments have less than 50% comminution
  ○ Type III: Cortices of both fragments have greater than 50% comminution
  ○ Type IV: Circumferential comminution

Tibia Plateau Fractures

- Classification: Schatzker
- Types: 6
  ○ Type I: Lateral plateau, split fracture
  ○ Type II: Lateral plateau, split depression fracture
  ○ Type III: Lateral plateau, depression fracture
  ○ Type IV: Medial plateau fracture
  ○ Type V: Bicondylar plateau fracture
  ○ Type VI: Bicondylar plateau fracture with metaphyseal separation from diaphysis

Ankle Fractures

- Classification: Lauge-Hansen
- Types: 4
  ○ Supination–adduction (SA)
    * Stage I: Transverse lateral malleolus fracture

* Stage II: Vertical medial malleolus fracture and transverse lateral malleolus fracture
  - Supination–external rotation (SER)
    * Stage I: Anterior tibiofibular ligament (ATFL) strain
    * Stage II: Oblique lateral malleolus fracture (anteroinferior to posterosuperior) and ATFL strain
    * Stage III: Posterior tibiofibular ligament disruption or posterior malleolus fracture, oblique lateral malleolus fracture, and ATFL strain
    * Stage IV: Transverse medial malleolus fracture or deltoid ligament rupture, posterior tibiofibular ligament (PTFL) disruption or posterior malleolus fracture, oblique lateral malleolus fracture, and ATFL strain
  - Pronation–abduction (PA)
    * Stage I: Transverse medial malleolus fracture or deltoid ligament rupture
    * Stage II: ATFL and transverse medial malleolus fracture
    * Stage III: High fibula fracture above syndesmosis with lateral comminution or butterfly fragment, ATFL, and transverse medial malleolus fracture
  - Pronation–external rotation (PER)
    * Stage I: Transverse medial malleolus fracture or deltoid ligament rupture
    * Stage II: ATFL and transverse medial malleolus fracture
    * Stage III: High oblique fibula fracture (anterosuperior to posteroinferior), ATFL, and transverse medial malleolus fracture
    * Stage IV: PTFL disruption, high oblique fibula fracture, ATFL, and transverse medial malleolus fracture

Fibular Fractures

* Classification: Danis-Weber (commonly known as Weber classification)

- Types: 3
  - Type A: Below the level of the tibial plafond
  - Type B: At the level of the tibial plafond
  - Type C: Above the level of the tibial plafond

Pilon or Plafond Fractures

- Classification: Rüedi and Allgöwer
- Types: 3
  - Type 1: Nondisplaced
  - Type 2: Displaced with minimal impaction or comminution
  - Type 3: Displaced with significant impaction and comminution

Calcaneus Fractures

- Classification: Sanders
- Types: 4
  - Type I: Nondisplaced
  - Type II: 2-part fractures of the posterior facet
  - Type III: 3-part fracture with central fragment depression
  - Type IV: 4-part articular fracture with significant comminution

Talar Neck Fractures

- Classification: Hawkins
- Types: 4
  - Type I: Nondisplaced
  - Type II: Talar neck fracture with subtalar subluxation/dislocation
  - Type III: Talar neck fracture with subtalar and tibiotalar dislocation
  - Type IV: Type III fracture with talonavicular sub luxation/dislocation

Navicular Body Fractures of the Foot

- Classification: Sangeorzan
- Types: 3
  - Type I: Navicular fractured into dorsal and plantar fragments

- o Type II: Navicular fractured into medial and lateral fragments
- o Type III: Comminution of fracture fragments and displacement

SPINE

Cervical Spine Fractures

- Odontoid fracture
- Classification: Anderson and D'Alonzo
- Types: 3
  - o Type I: Fracture at the tip of the odontoid
  - o Type II: Simple fracture at the junction of the neck and body
  - o Type IIA: Comminuted fracture at the junction of the neck and body
  - o Type III: Fracture below the odontoid waist into the body of C2
- Hangman's fracture
- Classification: Effendi
- Types: 3
  - o Type I: Nondisplaced fracture of pars interarticularis
  - o Type II: Displaced fracture of pars interarticularis
  - o Type IIA: Displaced fracture of pars interarticularis with avulsion of C2-3 intervertebral disc and posterior longitudinal ligament
  - o Type III: Displaced fracture of pars interarticularis and dislocation of C2-3 facet joints

Burst Fractures

- Classification: Denis
- Types: 5
  - o Type A: Both endplates fractured
  - o Type B: Superior endplate fractured
  - o Type C: Inferior endplate fractured
  - o Type D: Both endplates fractured with rotation
  - o Type E: Burst fracture with lateral flexion

Spinal Stability

- Classification: 3-column model of spinal stability
- Types: 3
  o Anterior column: Anterior longitudinal ligament, anterior half of vertebral body, and anterior annulus
  o Middle column: Posterior longitudinal ligament, posterior half of vertebral body, and posterior annulus
  o Posterior column: Pedicles, facets, facet capsules, lamina, supraspinous ligament, interspinous ligament, and ligamentum flavum

PEDIATRICS

Physeal Fractures

- Classification: Salter-Harris
- Types: 5
  o Type I: Transphyseal fracture
  o Type II: Transphyseal and metaphyseal fractures (Thurston-Holland fragment)
  o Type III: Transphyseal and epiphyseal fractures
  o Type IV: Transphyseal, metaphyseal, and epiphyseal fractures
  o Type V: Transphyseal crush injury
- Classification: Ogden
- Types: 4
  o Type VI: Perichondral ring injury at the physis periphery
  o Type VII: Epiphyseal fracture
  o Type VIII: Metaphyseal fracture
  o Type IX: Diaphyseal fracture

Supracondylar Humerus Fractures (Pediatric Population)

- Presentation: Extension type (95%), flexion type (5%)
- Classification: Gartland (extension type)
- Types: 3
  o Type I: Nondisplaced fracture (posterior fat pad sign)

- o   Type II: Displaced with intact posterior cortex
- o   Type III: Displaced with no cortical contact

Lateral Condyle Fractures of the Distal Humerus

- • Classification: Milch
- • Types: 2
  - o   Type I: Lateral condyle fracture lateral to the trochlea (Salter-Harris IV)
  - o   Type II: Lateral condyle fracture into the apex of the trochlea (Salter-Harris II)

Hip Fractures

- • Classification: Delbert
- • Types: 4
  - o   Type I: Transepiphyseal fracture
  - o   Type II: Transcervical fracture
  - o   Type III: Cervicotrochanteric fracture
  - o   Type IV: Intertrochanteric fracture

Tibial Tubercle Fractures

- • Classification: Watson-Jones
- • Types: 3
  - o   Type I: Fracture through secondary ossification center
  - o   Type II: Fracture through horizontal portion of tibial tubercle physis
  - o   Type III: Fracture through tibial tubercle and through tibial epiphysis

Tibial Spine Fractures

- • Classification: Meyers and McKeever
- • Types: 4
  - o   Type I: Minimal displacement
  - o   Type II: Intact posterior hinge
  - o   Type III: Complete displacement
  - o   Type IV: Comminuted

OPEN FRACTURE CLASSIFICATION

- Classification: Gustilo and Anderson
- Grades: 3
  - Grade I: <1-cm laceration, minimal muscle contusion, simple fracture
  - Grade II: >1-cm and <10-cm laceration with soft tissue damage, simple fracture with minimal comminution
  - Grade III:
    * Grade IIIA: >10-cm laceration, adequate soft tissue coverage of bone
    * Grade IIIB: Extensive soft tissue damage with periosteal stripping, requires soft tissue coverage
    * Grade IIIC: Vascular injury with fracture that requires repair
- Classification: Tscherne
- Grades: 4
  - Grade I: Small puncture wound and no contusions, low mechanism of injury
  - Grade II: Small laceration and contusions, moderate bacteria contamination
  - Grade III: Large laceration and extensive soft tissue damage, frequent neurovascular injury, heavy bacteria contamination
  - Grade IV: Incomplete or complete amputation

Traction Pin Placement

Traction pins are often placed in the lower extremities for the management of acetabular fractures, pelvic fractures, and femur fractures and for external fixators. If operative fracture fixation must be delayed for any reason, placing a traction pin prior to the operating room will stabilize the fracture and permit operative delay. The key point to remember with regards to approaches is that traction pins should be placed from the anatomic danger zone to a danger-free zone or to go from known to unknown. Enough weight should be placed on the traction pin to allow for adequate reduction of a fracture; for younger and more muscular individuals, more weight may be required, whereas the converse is often true for older individuals with less muscle mass. This section details the approaches to and perils of placing traction pins.

1. Distal femoral pin (Figure 16-1)

   a. Indications: Patients who have acetabular fractures, especially protrusio, may have a femoral traction placed in the distal femur. This reduces the femoral head to outside the pelvis, even though there is no bony acetabulum to contain the femoral head. A traction pin may also be used for traction to reduce an acetabular, pelvic, or hip fracture in the operating room.

   b. Approach: The femoral artery is located medially, as it travels through the Hunter canal. Thus, one should start medially and end the pin laterally.

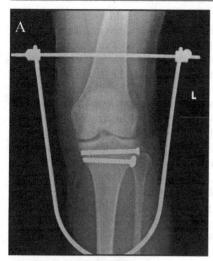

Figures 16-1. Distal femoral traction pin: (A) anteroposterior and (B) lateral.

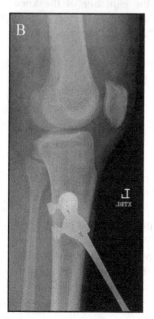

c. Procedure: The patient should be placed supine, with a bump under the knee to permit some flexion of the knee. One should mark approximately 2 to 3 cm proximal to the superior patella (or 2 to 3 finger breadths above the superior patella), which is just proximal to the adductor tubercle. The intersection between this point and the midpoint of the femoral shaft in the anteroposterior direction should be the starting point for the pin. This can be confirmed by using a radiopaque instrument to mark the location by fluoroscopy. A short longitudinal incision should be made and carried through the iliotibial band. The pin should be placed through the incision directly to bone. The anterior and posterior cortices of the femur should be palpated and the pin should be placed in the middle of the cortex. The pin should be drilled parallel to the joint line of the knee. Once the pin almost exits laterally, a short incision should be made over the tip of the pin. When the pin is out, the traction device should be ecured into place and radiographs should confirm placement.

d. Perils:

    i. Contraindications:

        1. Open injury over the location where a pin would be placed

        2. Femur fracture

    ii. A femoral traction pin placed too proximally may injure the femoral artery coming out of the Hunter canal.

    iii. A femoral traction pin placed too distally may injure the intercondylar notch of the femur.

    iv. Placing the pin with the knee in full extension may make it difficult for the patient to flex the knee if the pin is binding the iliotibial band.

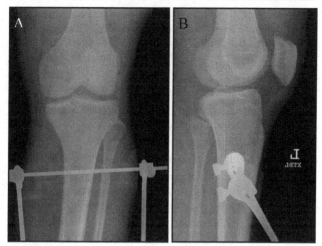

Figures 16-2. Proximal tibia traction pin: (A) anteroposterior and (B) lateral.

2. Proximal tibia pin (Figure 16-2)
   a. Indications: Patients who have femoral shaft fractures may have a tibial traction pin placed in the proximal tibia. Patients who have acetabular or pelvic fractures with ipsilateral damage to the femur may have a tibial traction placed in the proximal tibia.
   b. Approach: The peroneal nerve is located laterally as it travels around the fibular head. Thus, one should start laterally and end the pin medially.
   c. Procedure: The patient should be supine and the tibial tubercle should be palpated. The insertion of the pin is approximately 2 cm posterior and 2 cm distal from the tibial tubercle (approximately 2 finger breadths below the tibial tuberosity). Placement of the pin starting from the lateral leg can be confirmed by fluoroscopy. Once the pin

almost exits medially, a short incision should be
made over the tip of the pin. When the pin is out,
the traction device should be secured into place
and radiographs should confirm placement.

d. Perils:

i. Contraindications:

1. Open injury over the location where a pin
would be placed

2. Tibia fracture

3. Ligament injury to the ipsilateral knee

4. Pediatric population: Placing the pin in the
proximal tibia can damage the physis and
cause recurvatum injury to the bone.

ii. A tibial traction pin placed too proximally may
enter too much cancellous bone, which is weaker
than cortical bone.

iii. A tibial traction pin placed too proximally may
result in damage to the peroneal nerve.

iv. An incision placed too anteriorly may result in the
pin catching the posterior skin and may cause the
skin to gather.

3. Calcaneus pin (Figure 16-3)

a. Indications: Patients who have tibia or pilon
fractures, especially ones that require an external
fixation frame, may have a traction pin placed
through the calcaneus.

b. Approach: The posterior tibial nerve and artery,
medial calcaneal nerve, most posterior branch of
the lateral plantar nerve, and lateral plantar nerve
are located medially and travel inferior to the
medial malleolus. Thus, one should start medially
and end the pin laterally.

c. Procedure: The patient is placed supine and the
calcaneal tuberosity and the medial malleolus
should be palpated. A small incision should be
made approximately 3 cm below the medial malleolus in the quadrant posterior to the medial

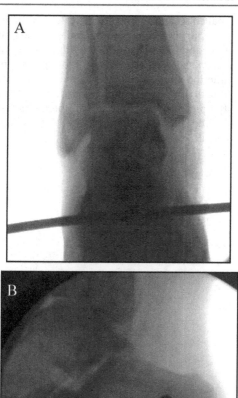

Figures 16-3. Calcaneus traction pin: (A) antero-posterior and (B) lateral.

malleolus and inferior to the calcaneal tuberosity. The pin should be placed parallel to the tibiotalar joint and can be confirmed by fluoroscopy. As the pin exits laterally, be sure to avoid placing the pin into the fibula. Once the pin almost exits laterally, a short incision should be made over the tip of the pin. When the pin is out, the traction device should be secured into place and radiographs should confirm placement.

d. Perils

  i. Contraindications:

    1. Open injury over the location where a pin would be placed

    2. Calcaneus fracture

Casts and Splints— Application and Usage

PRINCIPLES

1. Fracture stabilization: Stabilizing fractures with casts or splints can be for fracture treatment and for pain relief. Casts are circumferential and are often used to treat children with fractures. Splints are not circumferential, are used when limb edema is of concern, and are often used in adults for fresh fractures. Appropriate molding (3-point molding in casts) must be applied to ensure that fractures are adequately held in place.

2. Earlier mobilization: Stabilizing fractured extremities may allow the patient to ambulate on unaffected extremities earlier.

3. Improved function: Stabilizing an injured extremity may allow for improved use (eg, splinting a hand with wrist drop after a radial nerve injury).

4. Deformity correction: Casts may be used to correct extremity deformity, such as clubfoot casting (also known as Ponseti casting).

5. Prevent deformity progression: Casts may be used to decrease progression of certain diseases, such as scoliosis and neuromuscular imbalance conditions.

MATERIAL

1. Padding
   a. Webril (Covidien, Mansfield, Massachusetts): A padding made of dense cotton that can be rolled onto extremities. It has less motion within a cast or splint but has a tendency to become more wrinkled.
   b. Specialist (BSN Medical, Charlotte, North Carolina): A padding that is softer than Webril and is a cotton synthetic blend that contains wood fibers. It wrinkles less than Webril but slides more easily within casts or splints.
   c. Sof-Rol (BSN Medical, Charlotte, North Carolina): A padding made of rayon that is thicker than Webril, giving it higher tear resistance and great absorbency.
   d. Gore-tex (W. L. Gore & Associates, Incorporated, Flagstaff, Arizona): Waterproof material used in waterproof casts.

2. Wrap
   a. Plaster: A material composed of plaster of paris and crinoline that is used to immobile extremities, especially when there is a great deal of edema. Heat is released as the crystals interlock and the plaster hardens. Plaster may be rolled as a cast (especially if a reduction needs to be held) or applied in sheets as a splint. For splint application, approximately 8 to 12 sheets of plaster are used.
   b. Fiberglass: A material composed of fiberglass and polyurethane resin used in casting that becomes rigid with the addition of water or exposure to air.
   c. Ace/elastic wrap: A stretchy bandage used as a compressive dressing to hold a splint in place.
   d. Bias-cut stockinette: A cotton stocking with a single layer that can be used as a compressive dressing to hold a splint in place. Bias allows for more swelling than an Ace or elastic wrap.

3. Additional materials
   a. Tubular stockinette: A cotton stocking made of various diameters (2 to 12 inches) that can be used to cover an extremity prior to casting or may be fashioned into a sling if a sling is not available.
   b. Felt: A material composed of compressed fibers that can be used to pad bony prominences.
   c. Moleskin: A woven cotton fabric with a sticky surface that is used to pad the sharp edges of casts.

EQUIPMENT

1. Cast saw: An electric saw that uses an oscillating circular blade to cut through casts. because the saw blade oscillates, it does not cut skin and is the preferred method for removing casts.
2. Cast knife: A knife with a sharp blade that can be used to remove a cast.
3. Cast spreader: An instrument that can be placed between cut cast edges to spread the cast apart to facilitate removal.

CASTS AND SPLINTS: UPPER EXTREMITY

1. Coaptation splint (Figure 17-1)
   a. Application: humerus fractures.
   b. Description: A U-shaped splint that is placed from the base of the neck, wraps around the elbow, and ends under the axilla. The splint should be well padded within the axilla and the plaster should be proximal enough to ensure immobilization of the shoulder.
2. Long arm cast (Figure 17-2)
   a. Application: distal humerus, radial, and ulna fractures and immobilization after relocating elbow and radial head dislocations.

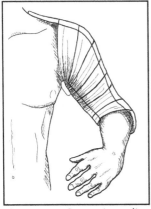

Figure 17-1. Coaptation splint.

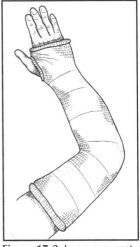

Figure 17-2. Long arm cast.

    b. Description: The arm is often placed at 90 degrees of flexion (supination and pronation are added based on injury). Padding and fiberglass wrap are placed from the proximal humerus to just proximal to the heads of the metacarpals. A mold is placed in the supracondylar humerus region, as well as between the radius and ulna.

3. Long arm splint (Figure 17-3)

    a. Application: distal humerus, radial, and ulna fractures, and immobilization after relocating elbow and radial head dislocations.

    b. Description: The arm is often placed at 90 degrees of flexion (supination and pronation are added based on injury) and padding is placed from the proximal humerus to just distal to the wrist. A posterior slab of plaster is applied from the humerus to the wrist. Side struts composed of 1-inch strips of plaster may be applied to improve the stability of the splint.

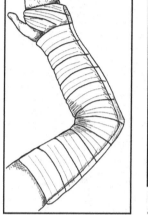
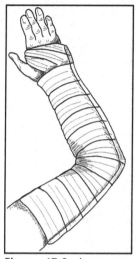

Figure 17-3. Long arm splint.

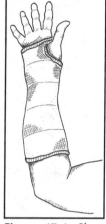

Figure 17-4. Short arm cast.

4. Short arm cast (Figure 17-4)

   a. Application: distal radius and ulna fractures, carpal bone fractures.

   b. Description: The wrist is positioned based on the injury. The wrist is placed in flexion and ulnar deviation for Colles fractures, in extension for Smith fractures, and neutral for carpal bone fractures. Padding and fiberglass wrap are placed from the proximal third forearm to proximal from the metacarpal heads.

5. Sugar tong (Figure 17-5)

   a. Application: radius and ulna fractures.

   b. Description: Padding is placed from the distal humerus to the heads of the metacarpals. The U-shaped plaster is wrapped from the dorsum of the hand, around the elbow, and into the palmar surface of the hand. Both the elbow and wrist joints are immobilized.

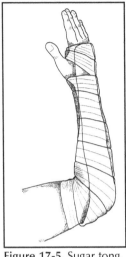

Figure 17-5. Sugar tong.

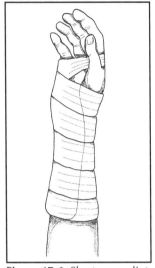

Figure 17-6. Short arm splint.

6. Short arm splint (Figure 17-6)
   a. Application: distal radius and ulna fractures.
   b. Description: This splint is often used in urgent care or emergency room settings for temporary immobilization. A plaster slab is placed volarly with the wrist in neutral and is wrapped in bias-cut stockinette or an elastic wrap.
7. Volar splint (Figure 17-7)
   a. Application: carpal, metacarpal, and phalangeal fractures.
   b. Description: The wrist is held in the intrinsic plus position or extension at the wrist, flexion at the metocarpophalangeal joint (60 to 70 degrees), and extension of the interphalangeal joints. Plaster is placed from the proximal third of the forearm to the distal tips of the fingers on the volar surface of the arm and hand.

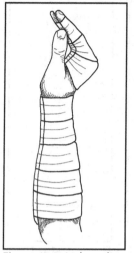 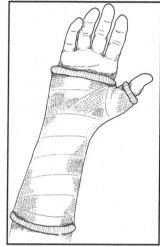

Figure 17-7. Volar splint.   **Figure 17-8.** Thumb spica cast.

8. Thumb spica cast (Figure 17-8)
   a. Application: thumb fractures (metacarpal and phalanges).
   b. Description: The thumb is extended and abducted, and padding and fiberglass wrap are applied from the proximal third of the forearm, past the wrist, and encapsulate the thumb.
9. Thumb spica splint (Figure 17-9)
   a. Application: thumb fractures (metacarpal and phalanges).
   b. Description: The thumb is extended and abducted, and padding and plaster are applied from the proximal third of the forearm, past the wrist, and encapsulate the thumb.
10. Ulnar gutter cast (Figure 17-10)
    a. Application: distal ulna fractures, and ring or small finger fractures (metacarpal and phalangeal).

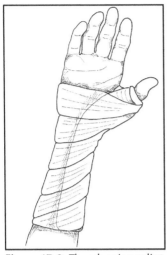 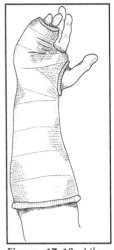

Figure 17-9. Thumb spica splint.   **Figure 17-10.** Ulnar gutter cast.

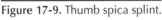

   b. Description: The ring and small fingers, as well as the wrist, are extended. Padding and fiberglass wrap are applied from the proximal third of the forearm to the distal ring and small fingers. The thumb, index, and long fingers remain free and are covered proximal to the metacarpal heads.

11. Ulnar gutter splint (Figure 17-11)
   a. Application: distal ulna fractures and ring or small finger fractures (metacarpal and phalangeal).
   b. Description: The ring and small fingers, as well as the wrist, are extended. Padding is applied from the proximal third of the forearm to proximal from the metacarpal heads and then is extended to enclose the distal ring and small fingers. A slab of plaster is applied on the lateral forearm and hand to encase the ring and small fingers.

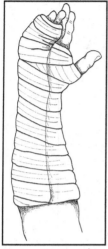

Figure 17-11. Ulnar gutter splint.

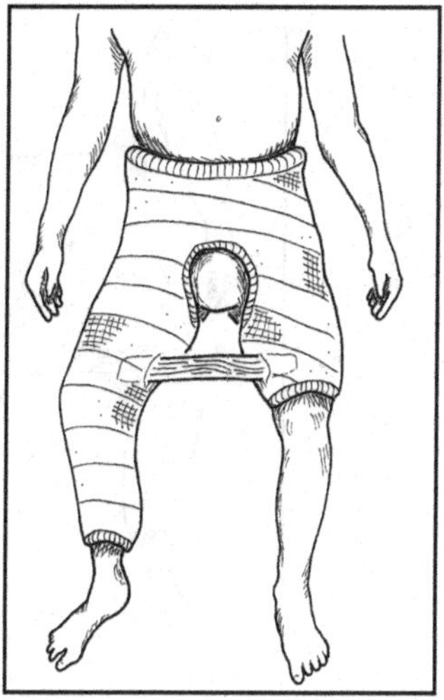

Figure 17-12. Half hip spica cast.

CASTS AND SPLINTS: LOWER EXTREMITY

1. Hip spica cast: half (Figure 17-12)
   a. Application: femur fractures (pediatric population).
   b. Description: Stockinette may be placed around the abdomen and bilateral legs. A stack of towels is often placed underneath the stockinette to enable room for chest wall expansion. Padding and fiberglass wrap are rolled from the abdomen, around both hips, down one leg (affected) proximal to the ankle, and down the contralateral (unaffected) leg proximal to the knee. A bar may be placed between both legs to provide stability. Care must be taken to cut out enough room for diaper placement and sharp cast surfaces should be covered with moleskin. The stack of towels should be removed after the cast is hardened.

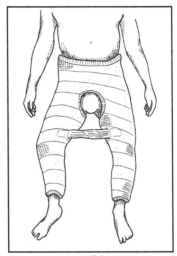

Figure 17-13. Full hip spica cast.

2. Hip spica cast: full (Figure 17-13)
   a. Application: femur fractures (pediatric population) that require more stability or bilateral femur fractures.
   b. Description: A stockinette may be placed around the abdomen and bilateral legs. A stack of towels is often placed underneath the stockinette to enable room for chest wall expansion. Padding and fiberglass wrap are rolled from the abdomen, around both hips, and down both legs proximal to the ankle. A bar should be placed between both legs to provide stability. Care must be taken to cut out enough room for diaper placement and sharp cast surfaces should be covered with moleskin. The stack of towels should be removed after the cast is hardened.

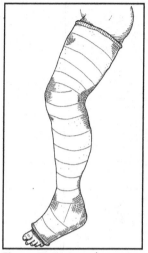
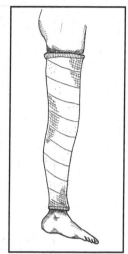

Figure 17-14. Long leg cast.

Figure 17-15. Cylinder cast.

3. Long leg cast (Figure 17-14)
   a. Application: distal femur, tibia, and ankle fractures and immobilization after relocating knee and ankle dislocations.
   b. Description: The knee is placed in 20 to 30 degrees of flexion and the ankle in 90 degrees of dorsiflexion. Padding and fiberglass wrap are applied from the proximal thigh by the groin and past the metatarsal heads. Extra padding is applied to the anterior knee and around the calcaneus, and minimal padding is applied to the anterior ankle. The toes are all left free. A mold is placed in the supracondylar femur region, the Achilles, and the arch of the foot.
4. Cylinder cast (Figure 17-15)
   a. Application: distal femur and proximal tibia fractures and immobilization after relocating knee dislocations.

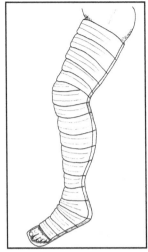

Figure 17-16. Long leg splint.

    b. Description: The knee is placed in extension. Padding and fiberglass wrap are applied from the proximal thigh by the groin and proximal to the medial and lateral malleoli. The ankle is not immobilized, and the cast may permit the patient to ambulate.

5. Long leg splint (Figure 17-16)

    a. Application: distal femur, tibia, and ankle fractures and immobilization after relocating knee and ankle dislocations.

    b. Description: The knee is placed in 20 to 30 degrees of flexion and the ankle in 90 degrees of dorsiflexion. Padding is applied from the proximal thigh by the groin to past the toes. A posterior slab of plaster is applied from the posterior thigh to the distal toes to ensure coverage of the metatarsals. The toes are all left free.

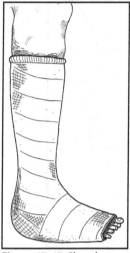

Figure 17-17. Short leg cast.

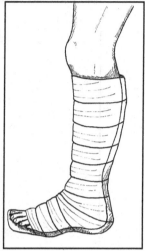

Figure 17-18. Short leg splint: posterior splint.

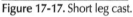

6. Short leg cast (Figure 17-17)
    a. Application: distal tibia, ankle, and foot fractures and immobilization after relocating ankle and foot dislocations.
    b. Description: The ankle is often placed in 90 degrees of dorsiflexion. Padding and fiberglass wrap are applied from distal to the tibial tubercle to past the metatarsal heads. Extra padding is applied around the calcaneus, and a mold is placed over the Achilles tendon and in the arch of the foot. The toes are all left free.
7. Short leg splint: posterior splint (Figure 17-18)
    a. Application: distal tibia, ankle, and foot fractures and immobilization after relocating ankle and foot dislocations.

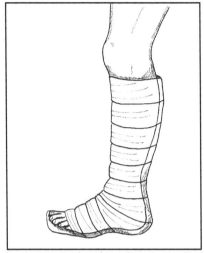

Figure 17-19. Short leg splint: team splint.

    b. Description: The ankle is often placed in 90 degrees of dorsiflexion. Padding is applied from distal to the tibial tubercle to past the toes. A posterior slab of plaster is applied to the posterior leg and is extended past the toes as a footplate. The toes are all left free.

8. Short leg splint: team splint (Figure 17-19)

    a. Application: distal tibia, ankle, and foot fractures and immobilization after relocating ankle and foot dislocations.

    b. Description: The ankle is often placed in 90 degrees of dorsiflexion. Padding is applied from distal to the tibial tubercle to past the toes. A posterior slab of plaster is applied to the posterior leg and is extended past the toes as a footplate. A U-shaped plaster slab is applied from the lateral leg, around the ankle, and ends on the medial leg. The toes are all left free. This splint offers more stability around the ankle.

Braces

SPINAL

- Soft cervical collar: A collar made of foam used to immobilize the cervical spine, either after injury or in the postoperative period (Figure 18-1).
- Hard cervical collar (eg, Philadelphia collar, Miami J collar [Ossur, Foothill Ranch, California], Aspen collar [Aspen Medical Products, Incorporated, Irvine, California]): A collar made of plastic with padding used to immobilize the cervical spine, either after injury or in the postoperative period (Figure 18-2).
- Minerva cervical orthosis (Lerman and Son Orthotics and Prosthetics, Beverley Hills, California): A brace used to treat scoliosis that includes the head and trunk, used for cervical spine fractures or spine deformities (Figure 18-3).
- Halo: A ring with 4 pins (adult) or 8 pins (child) that are fixed to the skull in order to maintain the alignment or stability of the cervical spine following surgery or trauma (Figure 18-4).
- Halo jacket: A halo with an attached vest that stabilizes the cervical spine to the trunk (see Figure 18-4).
- Hyperextension orthosis (eg, Jewett orthosis [Florida Brace Corporation, Winter Park, Florida]): A hyperextension trunk brace that provides a single 3-point force system via a sternal pad, a suprapubic pad, and a thoracolumbar pad that restricts forward flexion in the thoracolumbar area (Figure 18-5).

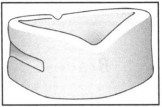

Figure 18-1. Soft cervical collar.

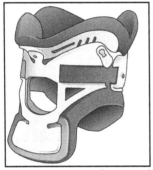

Figure 18-2. Hard cervical collar.

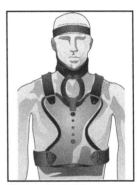

Figure 18-3. Minerva cervical orthosis.

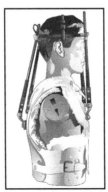

Figure 18-4. Halo and halo jacket.

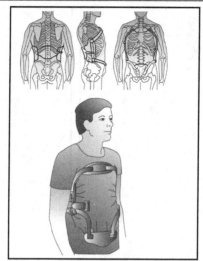

Figure 18-5. Hyperextension orthosis.

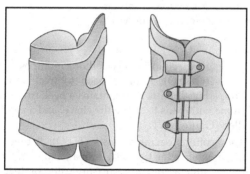

Figure 18-6. Boston scoliosis brace.

- Boston scoliosis brace (Boston Brace, Avon, Massachusetts): A molded chest and back brace used to control thoracic and lumbar scoliosis (Figure 18-6).

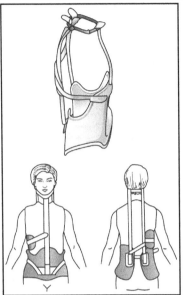

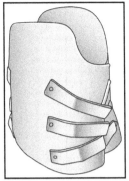

Figure 18-8. Thoracolumbosacral orthosis.

Figure 18-7. Milwaukee scoliosis cervicothoracolumbosacral orthosis.

- Milwaukee scoliosis cervicothoracolumbosacral orthosis (CTLSO): A brace used to treat adolescent idiopathic scoliosis that contains a neck ring, a trunk frame with pads to shape the curve, and a pelvic girdlen (Figure 18-7).
- Thoracolumbosacral orthosis (TLSO): A brace used to immobilize the thoracic, lumbar, and sacral spines, either after a fracture, postsurgically, or to correct scoliosis. May be a hard or soft brace (Figure 18-8).

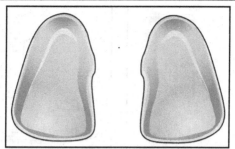

Figure 18-9. University of California Berkley Laboratory orthosis.

FOOT

- University of California Berkley Laboratory (UCBL) orthosis: An arch support that is molded to the foot designed to passively correct hindfoot or forefoot abnormalities in order to treat flexible flatfoot deformity (Figure 18-9).

- Controlled Action Motion boot (CAM; United States Manufacturing Company, Pasadena, California): A lower extremity brace that encircles the lower leg and looks like a boot. Patients may weight bear through the boot if instructed by their medical providers (Figure 18-10).

- Pressure-relief ankle–foot orthosis (PRAFO; Anatomical Concepts, Incorporated, Poland, Ohio): A static brace that keeps the foot in 90 degrees of dorsiflexion and provides padding to the heel to prevent pressure sores (Figure 18-11).

- Lace-up ankle brace (eg, Arizona brace [Custom Footwear, Incorporated, Mesa, Arizona]): A trademark lace-up ankle brace used to restrict motion at the ankle (Figure 18-12).

- Ankle–foot orthosis (AFO): An external device that controls the foot and ankle and can facilitate knee positioning and muscle response (Figure 18-13).

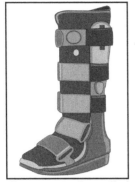

Figure 18-10. Controlled Action Motion boot.

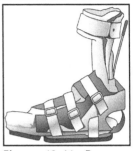

Figure 18-11. Pressure-relief ankle–foot orthosis.

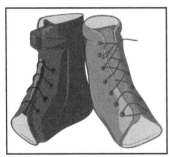

Figure 18-12. Lace-up ankle brace.

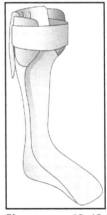

Figure 18-13. Ankle–foot orthosis.

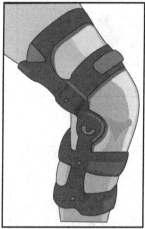

Figure 18-14. Hinged knee brace.

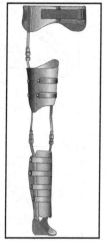

Figure 18-15. Hip–knee–ankle–foot orthosis.

LOWER EXTREMITY

- Hinged knee brace (eg, Bledsoe knee orthosis [Bledsoe, Grand Prairie, Texas], postoperative knee orthosis): A dynamic brace with adjustable ranges of motion that can be used to immobilize the knee after a fracture or surgery (Figure 18-14).

- Hip–knee–ankle–foot orthosis (HKAFO): A device to control all lower extremity segments. May be used after hip dislocations to prevent adduction and may be used after acetabular surgery to limit abduction and flexion (Figure 18-15).

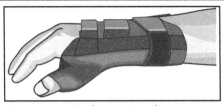

Figure 18-16. Cock-up wrist splint.

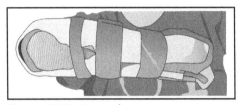

Figure 18-17. Munster brace.

UPPER EXTREMITY

- Cock-up wrist splint: A splint that immobilizes the wrist in an extended position. May be used in the setting of radial nerve injuries (Figure 18-16).
- Munster brace: A removable static brace to reduce forearm and wrist motion that is designed like a sugar tong splint, where the wrist and elbow are immobilized (Figure 18-17).
- Hinged elbow brace (elbow range of motion [ROM] brace): A dynamic brace with adjustable ranges of motion that can be used to immobilize the elbow after a fracture or surgery (Figure 18-18).
- Clavicle strap (figure 8 harness): A brace used to treat clavicle fractures that keep the shoulders extended (Figure 18-19).

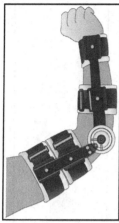

Figure 18-18. Hinged elbow brace.

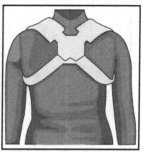

Figure 18-19. Clavicle strap.

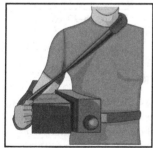

Figure 18-20. Abduction sling.

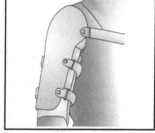

Figure 18-21. Sarmiento brace.

- Abduction sling (eg, Gunslinger orthosis [Sammons Preston, Bolingbrook, Illinois]): A sling with an attached pillow to keep the arm in abduction. Often used for the postoperative immobilization of shoulder after a rotator cuff repair (Figure 18-20).

- Sarmiento brace: A functional brace used to immobilize midshaft humerus fractures (Figure 18-21).

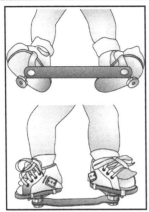

Figure 18-22. Abduction bar.

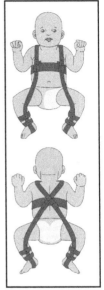

Figure 18-23. Pavlik harness.

PEDIATRICS

- Abduction bar (eg, Denis Brown bar, Fillauer bar, Tarso abduction bar): An orthopedic device used to position infant legs in abduction and external rotation. It is constructed by an aluminum bar with a pair of shoes fixed to the bar to position the feet (Figure 18-22).

- Pavlik harness: A brace used to treat congenital hip dislocations in an infant, where both legs are placed in the harness, the hips and knees are flexed, and the legs are abducted. May also be used to treat femur fracture in infants (Figure 18-23).

Analgesic Medications Commonly Used in Orthopedics

Pain management is paramount for treating musculoskeletal diseases and for postoperative care. A variety of narcotic and non-narcotic medications are frequently used in orthopedics. These medications can either be given by mouth (PO), intravenously (IV), intramuscularly (IM), subcutaneously (SC), and by rectum (PR). Intervals of medication administration range from every 4 hours (Q4h) to twice a day (BID), 3 times a day (TID), or as needed (PRN).

NONNARCOTIC MEDICATIONS

(see table)

Generic Name	Trade Name	Strengths	Common Dosages	Half-life (h)	Excretion
Acetaminophen	Tylenol	325, 500, 650; 120, 160/5 mL; 500/15 mL; 325, 650 PR	650 mg PO Q6h PRN	2 to 4	Liver
Celecoxib	Celebrex	50, 100, 200, 400	200 mg PO BID	11	Liver
Pregabalin	Lyrica	25, 50, 75, 100, 150, 200, 225, 300	150 mg PO BID	6	None
Gabapentin	Neurontin	100, 300, 400, 600, 800; 50/mL	300 mg PO TID	5 to 7	None
Tramadol	Ultram	50	50 mg PO Q6h PRN	6.3 to 7.9	Liver
Aspirin		81, 325, 500, 650; 60, 120, 200, 300, 600 PR	325 mg PO Q4h PRN 650 mg PO Q4h PRN	0.25 (aspirin) 2 to 6 (salicylate)	Liver, GI tract

Generic Name	Trade Name	Strengths	Common Dosages	Half-life (h)	Excretion
Ibuprofen	Advil/ Motrin	100, 200, 400, 600, 800; 50, 100 CH; 20, 40/mL	300 mg PO TID	2	Liver
Ketorolac	Toradol	10 PO, 60, 30, 15 IV/IM	10 mg PO Q4 to 6h 15/30 mg IV 30/60 mg IM	5	Liver
Diclofenac	Voltaren	25, 50, 75; 100 ER (extended release)	50 mg PO TID	2	Liver
Etodolac	Lodine	200, 300, 400, 500; 400, 500, 600 ER	300 mg PO BID 200 mg PO Q6 to 8h PRN	6.4	Liver
Indomethacin	Indocin	25, 50; 75 ER; 50 PR; IV	25 mg PO BID/TID	4.5	Liver
Meloxicam	Mobic	7.5, 15; 7.5/5 mL	7.5 mg PO daily	15 to 20	Liver
Naproxen		250, 375, 500; 375, 500; 125/5 mL	250 mg PO BID	12 to 17	Liver

Generic Name	Trade Name	Strengths	Common Dosages	Half-life (h)	Excretion
Piroxicam	Feldene	10, 20	20 mg PO daily	50	Liver
Salsalate		500, 750	1500 mg PO BID	1	Liver, GI tract

SHORT-ACTING ORAL NARCOTIC MEDICATIONS

Generic Name	Trade Name	Strengths	Common Dosages	Half-life (h)	Excretion	Notes
Codeine-acetaminophen	Tylenol #3	30/300, 60/300	30 mg PO Q4h PRN 60 mg PO Q4h PRN	2.5 to 3	Liver	Do not prescribe more than 4 g acetaminophen every day

Generic Name	Trade Name	Strengths	Common Dosages	Half-life (h)	Excretion	Notes
Hydrocodone-acetaminophen	Vicodin	5/500, 7.5/750 ES, (extra strength) 10/660 HP (high potency)	1 tab PO Q4h PRN	4	Liver	Do not prescribe more than 4 g acet-aminophen every day
Hydrocodone-acetaminophen	Norco	5/325, 7.5/325, 10/325	1 tab PO Q4h PRN	4	Liver	Less acet-aminophen per tablet compared to Vicodin
Oxycodone-acetaminophen	Percocet Roxicet	2.5/325, 5/325, 7.5/325, 7.5/500, 10/325, 10/650, 5/325/5 mL	1 tab PO Q4h PRN 5 mL PO Q4h PRN	4.5	Liver	Do not prescribe more than 4 g acet-aminophen every day

Generic Name	Trade Name	Strengths	Common Dosages	Half-life (h)	Excretion	Notes
Propoxyphene-acetaminophen	Darvocet	50/325, 100/500, 100/650	1 tab PO Q4h PRN	3.5 to 6.5	Liver	Withdrawn from the market due to increased cardiac arrhythmia risk
Hydromorphone	Dilaudid	2, 4, 8; 1/mL	2 mg PO Q4h PRN	2.5	Liver	
Morphine sulfate		15, 30; 2, 4, 20/mL sol; 5, 10, 20, 30 PR	1 tab PO Q4h PRN	2 to 4	Liver, GI tract	
Oxymorphone	Opana	5, 10; SC, IM, IV	10 mg PO Q4h PRN	7 to 11	Liver	

SHORT-ACTING INTRAVENOUS NARCOTIC MEDICATIONS

Generic Name	Trade Name	Strengths	Common Dosages	Half-life (h)	Excretion	Notes
Hydromorphone	Dilaudid	SC, IM, IV	0.1 to 1 mg IV Q3 to 6h PRN	2.3	Liver	Often used in patient-controlled anesthesia (PCA)
Morphine sulfate	Morphine	SC, IM, IV	1 to 2 mg IV Q3 to 6h PRN	2 to 4	Liver, GI tract	Often used in PCA
Meperidine	Demerol	SC, IM, IV	50 mg SC/IM Q4h PRN	2.5 to 4	Liver	
Fentanyl		IM, IV	50 to 100 mcg IV Q1 to 2h PRN	3.7	Liver	

LONG-ACTING NARCOTIC MEDICATIONS

Generic Name	Trade Name	Strengths	Common Dosages	Half-life (h)	Excretion	Notes
Morphine sulfate	MS Contin, Avinza, Kadian, Oramorph	15, 30, 60, 100, 200 ER	15 mg PO BID	2 to 4	Liver, GI tract	
Oxymorphone	Opana ER	5, 10, 20, 30, 40 ER	5 mg PO BID	7 to 11	Liver	
Oxycodone	Oxycontin	10, 15, 20, 30, 40, 60, 80 ER	10 mg PO BID	4.5	Liver	
Duragesic	Fentanyl patch	12, 25, 50, 75, 100 mcg/patch	1 patch Q72h	17	Liver	Transdermal administration
Methadone	Methadose, Dolophine	5, 10, 40; 5/5 mL, 10/5 mL, 10/mL sol; SC, IM, IV	15 mg PO daily	8 to 59	Liver	Titrate slowly to avoid withdrawal

Anticoagulation Medications Commonly Used in Orthopedics

Anticoagulation is imperative in the field of orthopedics for preventing deep vein thrombosis (DVTs), especially in lower extremity trauma and total joint arthroplasty. Prolonged periods of immobilization and reaming in the intramedullary canal can predispose a patient to a DVT. DVTs can form pulmonary emboli (PEs), which can be fatal. The following medications are the most commonly used anticoagulation medications in orthopedics that can be administered by mouth (PO), intravenously (IV), or subcutaneously (SC). Intervals of medication administration range from every 8 hours (Q8h) to twice a day (BID). Medications that are renally metabolized must be dose adjusted in patients with renal failure.

Chen AF, ed.
*Quick Reference Dictionary
for Orthopedics* (pp 355-358).

Generic Name	Trade Name	Method of Administration	Mechanism of Action	Prophylactic Dose	Therapeutic Dose	Half-Life (h)	Metabolism
Acetyl-salicylic acid	Aspirin	PO	Inhibits prostaglandin synthesis and prevents platelet aggregation	325 mg PO daily or BID	0.25 (aspirin)	2 to 6 (salicylate)	Liver and GI tract
Dabigatran	Pradaxa	PO	Inhibits thrombin	150 mg PO BID		12 to 17	Liver
Dalteparin	Fragmin	SC	Binds to antithrombin III (ATIII)	5000 U SC daily	200 U/kg SC daily	3 to 5	Liver
Desirudin	Iprivask	SC	Inhibits thrombin	15 mg SC BID		2	Renal

Generic Name	Trade Name	Method of Administration	Mechanism of Action	Prophylactic Dose	Therapeutic Dose	Half-Life (h)	Metabolism
Enoxaparin	Lovenox	SC, IV	Binds to ATIII	30 mg SC BID	1 mg/kg SC BID	4.5 to 7	Liver
Fondaparinux	Arixtra	SC	Selectively binds to ATIII	2.5 mg SC daily	(50 to 100 kg) 7.5 mg SC daily (>100 kg) 10 mg SC daily	17 to 21	Renal
Heparin		SC, IV	Binds to ATIII, inactivates thrombin	5000 U SC Q8h	18 U/kg/h IV	1.5	Liver
Rivaroxaban	Xarelto	PO	Factor Xa inhibitor	10 mg PO daily		5 to 9	Liver
Tinzaparin	Innohep	SC	Binds to ATIII	75 U/kg SC daily	175 U/kg SC daily	3 to 4	Unknown

Generic Name	Trade Name	Method of Administration	Mechanism of Action	Prophylactic Dose	Therapeutic Dose	Half-Life (h)	Metabolism
Warfarin	Coumadin	PO, IV	Inhibits vitamin K factors of coagulation (factors II, VII, IX, X proteins C and S)	2 to 5 mg PO daily	2 to 5 mg PO daily	20 to 60	Liver

Antibiotics Commonly Used in Orthopedics

There are multiple antibiotics available to use in the field of medicine, but some antibiotics are more commonly used than others. This is because orthopedic infections are mostly gram-positive organisms, specifically *Staphylococcus* and *Streptococcus* species of bacteria. Orthopedic management of infections, as in other parts of medicine, is often guided by the sensitivity of the organism based on cultures. However, cultures are not always available and may not always be positive. Patients are sometimes placed empirically on antibiotics for treatment, based on host factors and likely organisms. Below is a table of common antibiotics used for specific organisms and in specific situations. These medications can either be given by mouth (PO), intravenously (IV), or intramuscularly (IM). Intervals of medication administration range from every 6 hours (Q6h) to twice a day (BID), 3 times a day (TID), and 4 times a day (QID). Common organisms that are treated include *Staphylococcus aureus* (*S aureus*), methicillin-sensitive *S aureus* (MSSA), methicillin-resistant *S aureus* (MRSA), *Staphylococcus epidermidis* (*S epidermidis*), *Escherichia coli* (*E coli*), *Klebsiella pneumoniae* (*K pneumoniae*), and *Pseudomonas aeruginosa* (*P aeruginosa*). *Clostridium difficile* (*C difficile*) infections may be a consequence of antibiotic treatment.

Chen AF, ed.
*Quick Reference Dictionary
for Orthopedics (pp 359-366).*

Generic Name	Trade Name	Common Dosages	Mechanism of Action	Effective Against These Organisms	Notes
Amoxicillin	Amoxil	500 to 875 mg PO Q8h	Inhibits cell wall synthesis (β-lactam)	*Staphylococcus, Streptococcus,* and *E coli*	May lead to Stevens-Johnson syndrome, diarrhea, and *C difficile* colitis
Amoxicillin-clavulanate	Augmentin	875/125 mg PO Q8h	Inhibits cell wall synthesis and β-lactamases	Anaerobes, *Staphylococcus, Streptococcus,* and *E coli*	
Ampicillin		250 mg PO Q6h, 2 g IV Q4h	Inhibits cell wall synthesis	*Staphylococcus, Streptococcus,* and *Enterococcus*	
Ampicillin-sulbactam	Unasyn	1.5 to 3 g IV Q6h	Inhibits cell wall synthesis and β-lactamases	*Staphylococcus, Streptococcus, Enterobacter,* and anaerobes	

Generic Name	Trade Name	Common Dosages	Mechanism of Action	Effective Against These Organisms	Notes
Cefazolin	Ancef	1 to 2 g IV Q8h	First-generation cephalosporin, inhibits cell wall synthesis	*Staphylococcus* (MSSA) and *Streptococcus*	10% crossover reaction in patients with penicillin allergy, may lead to diarrhea and *C difficile* colitis
Cefepime	Maxipime	2 g IV Q12h	Fourth-generation cephalosporin, inhibits cell wall synthesis	*Pseudomonas aeruginosa, Enterobacter, Staphylococcus,* and *Streptococcus*	
Ceftazidime	Fortaz, Tazicef	2 g IV Q8 to 12h	Third-generation cephalosporin, inhibits cell wall synthesis	*Pseudomonas aeruginosa, Staphylococcus,* and *Streptococcus*	
Ceftriaxone	Rocephin	1 to 2 g IM/IV Q24h	Third-generation cephalosporin, inhibits cell wall synthesis	*Staphylococcus, Streptococcus, E coli,* and *K pneumoniae*	Also used to treat Lyme disease

Generic Name	Trade Name	Common Dosages	Mechanism of Action	Effective Against These Organisms	Notes
Cephalexin	Keflex	500 mg PO QID	First-generation cephalosporin, inhibits cell wall synthesis	*Staphylococcus* (MSSA) and *Streptococcus*	
Ciprofloxacin	Cipro	750 mg PO BID, 200 to 400 mg IV Q12h	Inhibits DNA gyrase and topoisomerase IV	*S aureus, S epidermidis, E coli, K pneumoniae,* and *P aeruginosa*	May predispose to tendon rupture, decreases seizure threshold
Clindamycin	Cleocin	450 mg PO Q8h, 600 mg IV Q6h	Binds to 50S ribosomal subunit, interferes with protein synthesis	*Staphylococcus, Streptococcus,* and anaerobes	
Daptomycin	Cubicin	4 to 6 mg/kg IV Q24h	Depolarizes bacterial membranes, inhibits protein/DNA/RNA synthesis	*Staphylococcus, Streptococcus,* and *Enterococcus*	May elevate liver function tests and lactate dehydrogenase, may lead to *C difficile* colitis

Generic Name	Trade Name	Common Dosages	Mechanism of Action	Effective Against These Organisms	Notes
Doxycycline	Vibramycin, Doryx, Oracea, Adoxa	100 mg PO Q24h	Inhibits protein synthesis	*Staphylococcus, Streptococcus, E coli,* and *K pneumoniae*	
Ertapenem	Invanz	1 g IM/IV daily	Inhibits cell wall synthesis	*Staphylococcus, Streptococcus, E coli,* and *K pneumoniae*	Not useful for MRSA and Enterococci
Fluconazole	Diflucan	400 mg PO daily	Inhibits cytochrome p450 and sterol C-14 alpha-demethylation	*Candida*	Hepatotoxic, may prolong QT interval
Gentamicin		1 mg/kg IV Q8h	Binds to 30S ribosomal subunit, interferes with protein synthesis	*Staphylococcus, Enterococcus, P aeruginosa, Proteus, Serratia*	Used in grade III open fractures, monitor for nephrotoxicity and ototoxicity

Generic Name	Trade Name	Common Dosages	Mechanism of Action	Effective Against These Organisms	Notes
Levofloxacin	Levaquin	750 mg PO BID	Inhibits DNA gyrase and topoisomerase IV	*S aureus, S epidermidis, E coli, K pneumoniae,* and *P aeruginosa*	May predispose to tendon rupture, decreases seizure threshold
Linezolid	Zyvox	600 mg PO/IV BID	Binds to 50S ribosomal subunit, interferes with protein synthesis	*Staphylococcus, Streptococcus,* and *Enterococcus*	Monitor complete blood count (may lead to myelo-suppression)
Meropenem	Merrem	1 g IV Q8h	Inhibits cell wall synthesis	*Staphylococcus Streptococcus, E coli, K pneumoniae*	
Metronidazole	Flagyl	500 mg IV/PO Q6 to 8h	Inhibits DNA synthesis	*Clostridium difficile,* anaerobes	May lead to peripheral neuropathy, ataxia, disulfram-like reaction
Nafcillin		12 g IV continuous daily	β-Lactamase resistant, inhibits cell wall synthesis	Penicillin-resistant *S aureus*	

Generic Name	Trade Name	Common Dosages	Mechanism of Action	Effective Against These Organisms	Notes
Oxacillin		12 g IV continuous daily	β-Lactamase resistant, inhibits cell wall synthesis	Penicillin-resistant *S aureus*, MSSA	
Penicillin		12 to 20 million U IV Q24h	Inhibits cell wall synthesis	Penicillin-sensitive *S aureus*, *Streptococcus*	Used in the presence of open fractures due to farm injuries
Piperacillin/ tazobactam	Zosyn	3.375 IV Q6h	Inhibits cell wall synthesis and β-lactamase	*Staphylococcus*, *Streptococcus*, and *K pneumoniae*	
Rifampin	Rifadin, Rimactane	300 mg PO BID	Inhibits DNA-dependent RNA polymerase	MRSA, *S epidermidis*, and *Mycobacterium*	May color body secretions orange, may lead to hepatotoxicity
Tetracycline	Sumycin	500 mg to 1 g PO BID	Inhibits protein synthesis	*Staphylococcus*, *Streptococcus*, *E coli*, and *K pneumoniae*	May cause peripheral and optic neuropathy, skin discoloration, and tooth discoloration in children

Generic Name	Trade Name	Common Dosages	Mechanism of Action	Effective Against These Organisms	Notes
Tigecycline	Tygacil	50 mg IV Q12h	Binds to 30S ribosomal subunit, interferes with protein synthesis	S aureus, MRSA, Streptococcus, and Acinetobacter baumannii	
Trimethoprim-sulfamethoxazole	Bactrim, Septra	1 DS PO BID	Inhibits folic acid synthesis and DNA synthesis	S aureus and E coli	May cause myelosuppression, elevated creatinine and potassium levels, and nephrotoxicity
Vancomycin	Vancocin	15 mg/kg IV Q12h	Inhibits cell wall and RNA synthesis	MRSA, coagulase-negative Staphylococcus	Monitor for red man syndrome and neutropenia, must monitor trough levels to prevent nephrotoxicity

APPENDIX 22

Imaging Modalities
in Orthopedics

Imaging is key for diagnostic and monitoring purposes in orthopedics. The following imaging modalities are used for different reasons.

X-Ray

X-rays are used as an initial screening tool for most musculoskeletal complaints, because they are the quickest and most cost-effective method of visualizing bones within the body. There are multiple views that can be obtained of different body parts:

1. Hand

   a. Anteroposterior (AP): visualize the carpal bones (especially the scaphoid)

   b. Lateral: visualize the lunate, pisiform, and metacarpals

   c. Oblique:

      i. Pronated oblique: visualize the scaphoid, triquetrum, body of hamate, scaphotriquetral, and trapezium-trapezoid joints

      ii. Supinated oblique: visualize the pisiform and pisotriquetral joint

2. Wrist

   a. AP: visualize the distal radius and distal ulna

   b. Lateral: visualize the distal radius tilt (volar inclination)

    c. Oblique: visualize the distal radioulnar joint (DRUJ)

3. Elbow

    a. AP: visualize the proximal radius (radial head and neck), proximal ulna, trochlea, and distal humerus

    b. Lateral: visualize elbow dislocations, radial head dislocations, the olecranon, and the humeral capitellum

4. Shoulder

    a. AP: visualize the glenohumeral joint

    b. Scapular Y: visualize proximal humerus fractures and scapular body fractures

    c. Axillary lateral: visualize shoulder dislocation, humeral head subluxation, glenohumeral joint

    d. Stryker notch view: visualize Hill-Sachs lesion

    e. West Point view: visualize bony Bankart lesion

    f. Supraspinatus outlet view: visualize subacromial impingement and acromial morphology

    g. Zanca view: visualize acromioclavicular joint

    h. Serendipity view: visualize sternoclavicular joint and medial one-third clavicle

    i. Garth view: visualize glenoid rim

    j. Grashey view: visualize glenohumeral joint for degenerative changes

5. Spine

    a. AP: visualize pedicles

    b. Lateral: visualize alignment of 3 columns (spondylolisthesis, fractures, etc)

    c. Supine, erect: assess spinal deformities with weight bearing views

    d. Flexion, extension: assess for spinal segmental instability

6. Pelvis

    a. AP: visualize the entire pelvis

      b. Judet (obdurator and iliac oblique): visualize the acetabulum

      c. Inlet/outlet views: visualize the pelvic ring

7. Hip

      a. AP: visualize abduction

      b. Lateral: visualize version of acetabulum

      c. Dunn view: visualize femoroacetabular impingement

8. Knee

      a. AP: visualize the femoral condyles, tibial plateau, and joint space (especially well assessed with flexion weight bearing posteroanterior view)

      b. Lateral: visualize the patella, distal and posterior femur, and proximal and posterior tibia

      c. Merchant view: visualize patellofemoral joint (eg, patellofemoral tilt)

      d. Sunrise view: visualize patellofemoral joint (eg, patellofemoral arthritis)

      e. Notch/tunnel view: visualize femoral notch, posterior femoral condyles, and intercondylar eminence of the tibia and assess for anterior cruciate ligament (ACL) injury

9. Ankle

      a. AP: visualize the tibiotalar joint, distal tibia, and distal fibula

      b. Lateral: visualize the tibiotalar joint, talocalcaneal joint, and bony anatomy (distal tibia, talus, and calcaneus)

      c. Mortise view: visualize the talar tilt, medial clear space (tibiotalar space), lateral clear space (between the fibula and talus), and interosseous clear space (between the tibia and fibula)

10. Foot

      a. AP: visualize metatarsals and Lisfranc joint

      b. Lateral: visualize the metatarsals, talus, calcaneus, and midfoot joints

c. Oblique: visualize the lateral metatarsals, the sinus tarsi, and midfoot articulations

d. Harris heel view: visualize the body of the calcaneus and the subtalar joint

MAGNETIC RESONANCE IMAGING

Magnetic resonance imaging (MRI) is nonionizing radiographical imaging that is often used to diagnose soft tissue diseases but can also be used in in bone imaging. For soft tissue, MRIs can be used to diagnose tendon and ligament tears, meniscal injuries, masses within the soft tissue, edema, effusions, and abscesses. For bone, an MRI can reveal an occult fracture, avascular necrosis, bone bruising, and osteomyelitis. MRIs are also used to assess other abnormalities in orthopedic conditions; for example, scoliosis patients with rapid curve progression, neurological symptoms, or a left thoracic curve.

There are multiple sequences that can be used to obtain different images in MRI. In T1-weighted sequences, fat appears bright, water appears dark, and bone appears white. In T2-weighted sequences, water appears bright, fat appears dark, and bone appears dark. In T2*-weighted sequences, the contrast is increased compared to T2 sequences but images take longer to acquire. Gadolinium (Gd), an intravenous or intra-articular MRI contrast agent, can be used to better assess abscesses.

As for contraindications, patients with cardiac pacemakers, ferrous implants, and brain aneurysm clips cannot get MRIs. Patients who have any chance of having metal in their eyes should get an orbital x-rays prior to MRIs to look for ferrous matter. Patients to be concerned about include iron workers, those exposed to shrapnel, and those who have tattoos that may have iron in the ink. Patients with renal disease may need to be pretreated prior to administering gadolinium contrast.

COMPUTED TOMOGRAPHY

Computed tomography (CT) scans are very useful for assessing bony morphology and fractures, because it is an x-ray imaging modality that produces 3-dimensional images. Bone is highly attenuated, which means that it appears white on CT scan. The following materials have decreasing amounts of attenuation on CT scan: bone, fat, water, soft tissue, and air (appears black on CT scans). CTs are especially useful for assessing articular fractures (pilon, tibial plateau, supracondylar femur, femoral head, glenohumeral, supracondylar humerus, and distal radius), fractures of the foot (especially calcaneus and talus fractures), and pelvic and acetabular fractures. For a more lifelike imaging of bone, the soft tissue can be windowed or leveled so that the bone is clearly visualized using 3-dimensional rendering. In cases where hardware is present, metal artifact correction can be performed to more clearly visualize the surrounding soft tissue. In cases when a MRI cannot be performed, a CT scan with contrast can be done (eg, CT myelogram to assess the spinal cord).

ULTRASONOGRAPHY

Ultrasound (US) has limited use in musculoskeletal imaging but can be used to diagnose conditions that are relatively superficial, such as abscesses near the surface of the skin and ligament and tendon pathologies. It can also be used for needle-guided aspirations and injections. Ultrasound has also been used to diagnose developmental dysplasia of the hip (DDH) and rotator cuff tears (RCTs).

For DDH, ultrasound is the preferred modality for evaluating the hip in patients who are 6 months of age or younger. After the age of 6 months, the capital femoral epiphysis begins to ossify, making it difficult to visualize the acetabulum. US allows for direct imaging of the cartilaginous portions of the hip that cannot be visualized on plain radiographs and permits dynamic study of the hip. A Barlow maneuver is performed on the hip and the following measurements are taken: (a) alpha angle: the angle between the acetabular roof and the vertical cortex of the ilium (normal value less than 60 degrees) and (b) beta angle: the angle formed between the triradiate cartilage and the vertical cortex of the ilium (more variable than the alpha angle). The Graf classification labels hip dysplasia into 4 types: (1) type I: normal, (2) type II: immature or mild dysplasia, (3) type III: dislocation, and (4) type IV: high dislocation.

For RCTs, ultrasound can visualize supraspinatus tears, as well as tendinosis, subacromial subdeltoid bursitis, subacromial impingement, adhesive capsulitis, calcific tendinitis, and greater tuberosity fractures. US can also be used to visualize and monitor surgical repairs.

ARTHROGRAPHY

An arthrogram, or arthrography, is performed to better visualize joints and the contents of joints. Dye is injected into a joint (see Appendix 14—Aspiration and Injection of and Around Joints), which provides contrast to the surrounding soft tissues. This permits clearer visualization of soft tissue structures, such as the labrum in the hip and shoulder. Injecting contrast into a joint under fluoroscopy permits one to examine whether the dye extravasates, which would indicate that there is an intra-articular fracture. An arthrogram is also an ideal imaging modality for visualizing cysts and joint capsules.

BONE SCINTIGRAPHY

A bone scan, or bone scintigraphy, is a nuclear scanning study that injects a small dose of radioactive marker that collects in bone. The image is then captured by a gamma camera, and areas of greater bone turnover will be visualized. Conditions that are diagnosed by bone scan include bone tumors (especially metastatic cancer), osteomyelitis, fractures, and implant loosening. Though bone scans are sensitive, they are not very specific.

In a 1-phase bone scan, patients are injected with the radioactive marker and are imaged 2 to 3 hours later. Three-phase bone scans are used to evaluate for osteomyelitis or fractures; images acquired in the first- and second-phase images are taken within the first 30 to 70 minutes and the third phase is taken 2 to 3 hours later. Patients may be scanned up to 24 hours later.

Another variation of this scan is the white blood cell (WBC) scan, which is also known as an indium scan, Ceretec scan, or inflammatory scan. For this scan, WBCs are removed from the patient's blood and tagged with indium-111. The WBCs are returned into the patient 2 to 3 hours later and the patient is scanned 6 to 24 hours later. This scan can localize areas of increased WBC cells that are indicative of infection or inflammation.

POSITRON EMISSION TOMOGRAPHY

A positron emission tomography (PET) scan is a nuclear medicine imaging technique that uses positron-emitting radionuclide ligands to detect functional physiology through imaging of metabolically active areas. A common ligand that is used is fluorodeoxyglucose (FDG), an analog of glucose, which is used to identify sections of the body that have increased metabolic activity. PET may be used in orthopedics to identify tumor locations and determine muscle activity, especially of deeper muscles. PET can be combined with another imaging modality (eg, MRI or CT scan) for ED localization of metabolic activity. However, combined PET/CT scans have substantially more radiation than PET or CT scans alone.

Nerve Conduction Studies and Electromyography

TESTS

Nerve conduction studies (NCS) and electromyography (EMG) are 2 different tests that assess the electrical activity of muscles by assessing the motor and sensory nerves and the muscles, respectively. NCS are less invasive and are often used as a first-line test for conditions such as carpal tunnel syndrome. EMGs are more invasive and are useful for assessing for muscle disease. Both tests should not be conducted in the acute injury phase and should be delayed 7 to 21 days after injury when denervation occurs.

NERVE CONDUCTION STUDIES

1. Usage: NCS are used to evaluate weakness or paresthesia in the upper and lower extremities. Conditions that are often diagnosed include carpal tunnel syndrome (CTS), peripheral neuropathy, ulnar neuropathy, and Guillian-Barré syndrome.

2. Procedure: Needles are placed at 2 points in a nerve trunk so that all of the motor or sensory axons are stimulated when an electrical pulse is applied (0.1 to 0.5 milliseconds, 60 to 300 V). The latency is the time for the electrical impulse to travel from the site of stimulation to the needle that is measuring the impulse. Conduction velocity is determined by the distance traveled between the 2 needles divided by the difference in latency between the 2 points.

Chen AF, ed.
*Quick Reference Dictionary
for Orthopedics (pp 374-376).*

3. Results: There are 4 different tests: motor NCS, sensory NCS, F-wave study, and H-reflex study. The 2 most commonly used tests are motor and sensory NCS.

   a. Motor NCS: A peripheral nerve is stimulated and the muscle response is recorded. A normal motor conduction velocity is greater than 45 m/s in the arm and is greater than 40 m/s in the leg. This can vary with temperature—a 1°C increase in temperature can result in a conduction velocity increase by 2.4 m/s. Conduction velocity is also faster in proximal segments of a limb compared to distal segments. Motor latency is normally less than 5 milliseconds in distal limbs but less than 7 milliseconds in the peroneal and posterior tibial nerves.

   b. Sensory NCS: A peripheral nerve is stimulated and the sensory nerve response is recorded. A normal sensory nerve conduction velocity in the arm is greater than 35 m/s. Sensory latency is normally less than 4 milliseconds, and latency greater than 6 milliseconds is considered severe. Sensory NCS is a more sensitive test for detecting carpal tunnel syndrome.

ELECTROMYOGRAPHY

1. Usage: EMGs are used to measure the electrical activity from skeletal muscles or lower motor neuron diseases. Conditions that are often diagnosed include myasthenia gravis and amyotrophic lateral sclerosis.

2. Procedure: Three electrodes are used to detect electrical activity from a muscle. One electrode is a recording electrode, another is an indifferent electrode that subtracts background noise, and the last is a ground electrode. Muscles are measured at rest and when contracting. Measurements are described in action potential (voltage, V) and the frequency of the muscle

motor unit firing (hertz, Hz). The waves are described by size, shape, amplitude, and frequency. Depending on the muscle type, normal EMG potentials range from 50 µV to 30 mV and frequency ranges from 7 to 20 Hz.

3. Disease results: The following disease classes have characteristic EMG findings:

   a. Neuropathic disease

      i.   Action potential amplitude: increased (due to reinnervation)

      ii. Action potential duration: increased

      iii. Number of motor units: decreased

   b. Myopathic disease

      i.   Action potential duration: decreased

      ii. Area to amplitude ratio: decreased

      iii. Number of motor units: decreased

4. EMG results: The following EMG findings are indicative of certain disease states:

   a. No action potential: Diagnosis = Complete nerve lesion

   b. Small polyphasic units: Diagnosis = Primary muscle disease

   c. Pseudomyotonic discharge: Diagnosis = Polymyositis, alcoholic neuropathy

   d. Myotonic voltage discharge: Diagnosis = Myotonia congenita

   e. Nascent motor unit: Diagnosis = Regenerating nerve

   f. Positive sharp waves, fibrillation potentials: Diagnosis = Partially denervated muscle

   g. Polyphasic motor unit voltages: Diagnosis = Chronic denervation

Research in Orthopedics

1. Timing of studies
   a. Prospective: A study that collects data forward in time.
   b. Retrospective: A study that collects data from the past.
2. Types of studies (see table on page 378)
   a. Experimental
      i. Randomized controlled trial (RCT): A prospective study in which patients are randomly assigned to a specific intervention and the outcomes are compared. This is the gold standard for clinical trials.
   b. Observational
      i. Cohort study: A longitudinal study in which a group of individuals with a shared characteristic are followed for a period of time to determine the risk of developing a certain condition.
         1. Prospective cohort study: A study in which the patient populations are defined before following the patients longitudinally.
         2. Retrospective cohort study: A study in which the patient populations are defined after the data have been collected.

Chen AF, ed.
*Quick Reference Dictionary
for Orthopedics* (pp 377-385).

TYPE OF STUDY

	Therapeutic	Prognostic	Diagnostic	Economic or Decision Analysis
Level I	RCT or systematic review on RCT	Prospective study or systematic review of Level I studies	Testing of established diagnostic criteria in consecutive patients or systematic review of Level I studies	Provides clinically sensible costs, values are obtained from multiple studies, multi-way sensitivity analysis performed, or systematic review of Level I studies
Level II	Prospective cohort studies, lower quality RCT, and systematic review of Level II studies	Retrospective study, study of untreated controls from RCT, and systematic review of Level II studies	Development of diagnostic criteria in consecutive patients or systematic review of Level II studies	Provides clinically sensible costs, values are obtained from limited studies, multi-way sensitivity analysis performed, or systematic review of Level II studies
Level III	Case-control studies, retrospective cohort studies, and systematic review of Level III studies		Diagnostic studies in nonconsecutive patients or systematic review of Level III studies	Clinically limited costs and poor estimates; or systematic review of Level III studies

TYPE OF STUDY

	Therapeutic	Prognostic	Diagnostic	Economic or Decision Analysis
Level IV	Case series	Case series	Case-control studies	Studies without sensitivity analysis
Level V	Expert opinion	Expert opinion	Expert opinion	Expert opinion

    ii. Case-control study: A study in which a group of patients with a condition is compared to a group that does not have the condition.

    iii. Cross-sectional study: A descriptive study in which an entire population is analyzed at a certain point in time.

    iv. Case series: A study in which individual patients are described.

3. Levels of evidence (see table on page 381)

4. Error

    a. Alpha (α): The probability of incorrectly rejecting the null hypothesis (type I error, false positive). Often set to 5%.

    b. Beta (β) = Power: The probability of incorrectly retaining the null hypothesis (type II error, false negative). Often set to 80%.

5. Sample size: An adequate number of subjects must be included in a study in order to achieve sufficient statistical power. This may be difficult in studies examining rare conditions. Sample size calculations are based on the desired confidence interval (or the alpha value), the power level, and the value of the variable of interest based on previous studies.

6. Types of variables

    a. Continuous: A quantitative variable that can take on any number (eg, age and weight).

    b. Discrete: A quantitative variable that can only take on whole numbers (eg, number of surgeries).

    c. Nominal: A categorical variable (eg, gender: male/female, laterality: left/right).

    d. Ordinal: A variable that is rank ordered (eg, American Society of Anesthesiologists [ASA] physical status classification).

    e. Interval: A variable that is rank ordered and is separated by the same interval (eg, temperature in Fahrenheit or Celsius) to permit numerical comparisons between values.

TYPE OF STUDY

	Therapeutic	Prognostic	Diagnostic	Economic or Decision Analysis
Level I	RCTs or systematic review on RCTs	Prospective study or systematic review of Level I studies	Testing of established diagnostic criteria in consecutive patients or systematic review of Level I studies	Provides clinically sensible costs, values are obtained from multiple studies, multiway sensitivity analysis performed; or systematic review of Level I studies
Level II	Prospective cohort studies, lower quality RCTs, and systematic review of Level II studies	Retrospective study, study of untreated controls from RCT, and systematic review of Level II studies	Development of diagnostic criteria in consecutive patients or systematic review of Level II studies	Provides clinically sensible costs, values are obtained from limited studies, multiway sensitivity analysis performed; or systematic review of Level II studies
Level III	Case-control studies, retrospective cohort studies, and systematic review of Level III studies		Diagnostic studies in nonconsecutive patients or systematic review of Level III studies	Clinically limited costs and poor estimates; or systematic review of Level III studies
Level IV	Case series	Case series	Case-control series	Studies without sensitivity analysis
Level V	Expert opinion	Expert opinion	Expert opinion	Expert opinion

   f. Ratio: A variable that is rank ordered, can be compared between values, and also has an absolute zero point (eg, temperature in Kelvin).

7. Commonly used statistical tests

   a. Student's t test: Test to compare means between 2 samples that are normally distributed (may be independent one-sample t test, independent 2-sample t test, or dependent t test for paired samples).

   b. Analysis of variance (ANOVA): Test to compare 3 or more groups of continuous variables that are normally distributed.

   c. Regression: Test where the outcome is predicted by a model (linear, multiple, logistic) as a function of other variables/predictors.

   d. Analysis of covariance (ANCOVA): Test that combines regression and ANOVA for continuous variables, which tests if certain factors have an affect on the outcome if certain variables are removed.

   e. Pearson's chi-square test: Test to compare 2 or more groups of nominal variables.

   f. Fisher's exact test: Test to compare 2 groups of nominal variables that have cell frequencies that are 5 or less.

   g. Mann-Whitney U test (Wilcoxon rank-sum test): Test to compare 2 groups of continuous or ordinal variables that do not follow a normal distribution.

   h. Wilcoxon signed-rank test: Paired test to compare 3 or more groups of continuous or ordinal variables that do not follow a normal distribution.

   i. Kruskal-Wallis test: Test to compare 3 or more groups of continuous or ordinal variables that do not follow a normal distribution.

   j. Friedman's test: Paired test to compare 3 or more groups of continuous or ordinal variables that do not follow a normal distribution.

k. McNemar's test: Paired test to compare 2 nominal variables.

l. Cochran's Q test: Paired test to compare 3 or more nominal variables.

m. Log-rank test: Test to compare survival in independent groups.

n. Conditional logistic regression: Test to compare survival in paired groups.

8. Statistical outputs

a. Sensitivity: Percentage of subjects that are true positives, rules a disease out.

b. Specificity: Percentage of subjects that are true negatives, rules a disease in.

c. Likelihood ratio: Probability of true positives divided by true negatives.

d. Positive predictive value (PPV): Probability of having a disease when the test result is positive.

e. Negative predictive value (NPV): Probability of not having a disease when the test result is negative.

f. Receiver operating curve (ROC): Area calculated under the curve demonstrating a test's performance as related to the true positive (sensitivity) and false positive (1 − specificity) rates.

g. P value: The probability of determining whether the obtained results are by chance or if the null hypothesis is true. As a measure of statistical significance, a P value that is less than the alpha value (.05) is often considered statistically significant.

h. Confidence interval (CI): The percentage probability that the true value lies within a range of values, often 95%.

i. r^2: In linear regressions, the coefficient of determination is the square of the correlation coefficient (r) that quantitates the correlation between variables. Stronger correlations approach $r^2 = 1$.

j. Odds ratio (OR): The ratio of the odds of having a disease in the case group to the odds of having a disease in the control group. Can be calculated in cross-sectional, retrospective case-control, or retrospective cohort studies.

k. Relative risk (RR): The incidence of a disease in the experimental cohort divided by the incidence of a disease in the control cohort. Can only be calculated from prospective cohort studies.

l. Absolute risk reduction (ARR): The difference in risk of adverse events when comparing experimental and control groups in a study.

m. Relative risk reduction (RRR): The proportion of reduction in adverse events when comparing experimental and control groups in a study.

n. Number needed to treat (NNT): The number of patients that need to be treated to obtain 1 additional positive outcome.

9. Bias: Favoring an outcome due to random or systematic statistical sampling or testing error. Bias can be minimized by randomizing studies, blinding the data collectors, and matching patients. Though there are many sources of bias, the main sources are highlighted below:

a. Selection bias: Comparison of dissimilar groups

   i. Selection bias: Selection of a nonrandom group of individuals within a population.

   ii. Volunteer bias: When a subject volunteers or is referred to participate in a study, he or she may be more motivated than others.

   iii. Nonrespondent bias: When a subject does not respond to a survey request, decreased follow-up rate.

   iv. Attrition bias: Bias from the loss of participants.

   v. Undercoverage bias: When a certain sample of the population is underrepresented in the study.

b. Measurement bias

    i. Lead time bias: Bias where the perceived survival time increases due to earlier diagnosis, not due to an effect on the outcome of a disease.

    ii. Instrument bias: Calibration errors that lead to inaccurate measurements.

    iii. Insensitive measure bias: When a measurement tool is not sensitive enough to detect differences in the variable being studied.

    iv. Expectation bias: When observers measure data with an expected outcome, because the patients are not masked and the observers are not blinded.

    v. Recall bias: Bias due to subjects' recall of past events.

    vi. Attention bias: Bias due to subject's awareness of being a part of a study.

    vii. Leading question bias: Wording a question to favor one response over another. Also known as interviewer bias.

c. Intervention bias

    i. Contamination bias: When the control group inadvertently receives exposure to the intervention.

    ii. Co-intervention bias: When subjects are receiving other interventions simultaneously with the study intervention.

    iii. Timing bias: A study duration that is too short to notice a difference or too long, where improvement is not due to study intervention but rather to maturation.

    iv. Compliance bias: When subjects do not adhere to the study intervention.

    v. Withdrawal bias: When subjects withdraw from the study.

    vi. Proficiency bias: When the interventions are not equally administered to subjects due to technical differences among personnel.

Orthopedic Associations

GENERAL SOCIETIES

AAOS: American Academy of Orthopaedic Surgeons
AOA: American Orthopaedic Association
ORS: Orthopaedic Research Society

SUBSPECIALTIES

AAHKS: American Association of Hip and Knee Surgeons
AANA: Arthroscopy Association of North America
ACSM: American College of Sports Medicine
AOFAS: American Orthopaedic Foot and Ankle Society
AOSSM: American Orthopaedic Society for Sports Medicine
ASES: American Shoulder and Elbow Surgeons
ASIA: American Spinal Injury Association
ASSH: American Society for Surgery of the Hand
MTS: Musculoskeletal Tumor Society
NASS: North American Spine Society
OTA: Orthopaedic Trauma Association
POSNA: Pediatric Orthopaedic Society of North America
SAS: Spine Arthroplasty Society
SRS: Scoliosis Research Society

INTERNATIONAL

FIMS: International Federation of Sports Medicine
ICJR: International Congress on Joint Reconstruction

Chen AF, ed.
*Quick Reference Dictionary
for Orthopedics (pp 386-390).*
© 2012 Taylor & Francis Group.

ICRS: International Cartilage Repair Society

ICSES: International Congress of Shoulder and Elbow Surgery

IFFAS: International Federation of Foot and Ankle Surgeons

IMRRS: International Musculoskeletal Regeneration and Research Society

ISAKOS: International Society of Arthroscopy, Knee Surgery and Orthopaedic Sports Medicine

ISFR: International Society for Fracture Repair

ISHA: International Society for Hip Arthroscopy

ISMSP: International Sports Medicine Science and Performance

ISTA: International Society for Technology in Arthroplasty

SICOT: International Society of Orthopaedic Surgery and Traumatology

REGION-SPECIFIC SOCIETIES

APAS: Asia Pacific Arthroplasty Association

APOA: Asia Pacific Orthopaedic Association

APOSSM: Asia Pacific Orthopaedic Society for Sports Medicine

EFAS: European Foot and Ankle Society

EFORT: European Federation of National Associations of Orthopaedics and Traumatology

EFOST: European Federation of National Associations of Orthopaedic Sports Traumatology

EORS: European Orthopaedic Research Society

EPOS: European Paediatric Orthopaedic Society

ESSKA: European Society of Sports Traumatology, Knee Surgery and Arthroscopy

ESSSE/SECEC: European Society for Surgery of Shoulder and Elbow

ETS: European Trauma Society

FESSH: Federation of the European Societies for the Surgery of the Hand

COUNTRY-SPECIFIC SOCIETIES

AOS: Austrian Orthopaedic Society
AOTRF: Association of Orthopaedic and Trauma Surgeons of the Russian Federation
AuOA: Australian Orthopaedic Association
BASEM: British Association of Sports and Exercise Medicine
BASK: British Association for Surgery of the Knee
BASS: British Association of Spine Surgeons
BCSS: British Cervical Spine Society
BESS: British Elbow and Shoulder Society
BHS: British Hip Society
BOA: British Orthopaedic Association
BOFAS: British Orthopaedic Foot and Ankle Society
BOOS: British Orthopaedic Oncology Society
BORS: British Orthopaedic Research Society
BOS: Bangladesh Orthopaedic Society
BOSA: British Orthopaedic Specialists Association
BOSTA: British Orthopaedic Sports Trauma Association
BOTA: Bulgarian Orthopaedics and Traumatology Association
BSCOS: British Society for Children's Orthopaedic Surgery
BSS: British Scoliosis Society
BSSH: British Society for Surgery of the Hand
BTS: British Trauma Society
BulOrtho: Bulgarian Orthopaedic Association
BVOT: Belgian Orthopaedic and Trauma Society
ChOA: Chinese Orthopaedic Association
COA: Canadian Orthopaedic Association
CyOA: Cyprus Orthopaedic Association
DOS: Dutch Orthopaedic Society
DuOA: Dutch Orthopaedic Association
EBJIS: European Bone and Joint Infection Society
EOA: Egyptian Orthopaedic Association
ESTES: European Society of Trauma and Emergency Surgery
FOA: Finnish Orthopaedic Association
GOS: German Orthopaedic Society
HAOST: Greek Orthopaedic Association

HKOA: Hong Kong Orthopaedic Association
HOS: Hungarian Orthopaedic Society
HuOA: Hungarian Orthopaedic Association
HUOT: Croatian Orthopaedic and Traumatology Association
IAA: Indian Arthroscopy Association
IcOA: Icelandic Orthopaedic Association
IndoOA: Indonesian Orthopaedic Association
IOACON: Indian Orthopaedic Association
IrOA: Iranian Orthopaedic Association
IrOA: Irish Orthopaedic Association
IsOA: Israeli Orthopaedic Association
JOA: Japanese Orthopaedic Association
JOA-MST: Musculoskeletal Tumour Meeting of Japanese Orthopaedic Association
JOA-ORS: Japanese Orthopaedic Association–Orthopaedic Research Society
KOA: Korean Orthopaedic Association
MOA: Malaysian Orthopaedic Association
MOA: Mexican Orthopaedic Association
NOA: Nepal Orthopaedic Association
NZOA: New Zealand Orthopaedic Association
PhilOrtho: Philippine Orthopaedic Association
POOA: Polish Orthopaedic Association
POS: Polish Orthopaedic Society
POSI: Paediatric Orthopaedic Society of India
ROS: Russian Orthopaedic Society
SAOA: South African Orthopaedic Association
SAROA: Saudi Arabian Orthopaedic Association
SCHOT: Chilean Orthopaedic Association
SECOT: Spanish Orthopaedic Society
SGOSSO: Swiss Orthopaedic Association
SOA: Singapore Orthopaedic Association
SOROT: Romanian Orthopaedic Association
SOS: Swedish Orthopaedic Society
SyOA: Syrian Orthopaedic Association
TaiOA: Taiwanese Orthopaedic Association
TOA/RCOST: Thailand Orthopaedic Association
TOTBID: Turkish Orthopaedic Association

TSTAK: Turkish Sports Traumatology Arthroscopy and Knee Surgery

VenOA: Venezuelan Orthopaedic Association

Printed in the United States
by Baker & Taylor Publisher Services

Printed in the United States
by Baker & Taylor Publisher Services